Natural Antibiotics

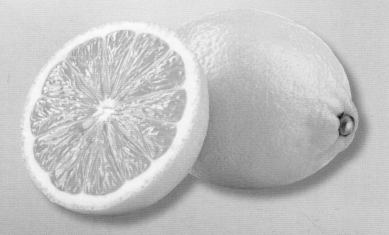

Publications International, Ltd.

Photography: Alamy, Gil Nelson, Claudio Pistilli, and Shutterstock.com

Louis Weber, CEO
Publications International, Ltd.
8140 Lehigh Avenue
Morton Grove, IL 60053

Permission is never granted for commercial purposes.

ISBN: 978-1-64030-874-9

Manufactured in China.

8 7 6 5 4 3 2 1

This publication is only intended to provide general information. The information is specifically not intended to be a substitute for medical diagnosis or treatment by your physician or other healthcare professional. You should always consult your own physician or other healthcare professionals about any medical questions, diagnosis, or treatment. (Products vary among manufacturers. Please check labels carefully to confirm that the products you use are appropriate for your condition.)

The information obtained by you from this publication should not be relied upon for any personal, nutritional, or medical decision. You should consult an appropriate professional for specific advice tailored to your specific situation. PIL makes no representation or warranties, express or implied, with respect to your use of this information.

In no event shall PIL or its affiliates or advertisers be liable for any direct, indirect, punitive, incidental, special, or consequential damages, or any damages whatsoever including, without limitation, damages for personal injury, death, damage to property or loss of profits, arising out of or in any way connected with the use of any of the above-referenced information or otherwise arising out of use of this publication.

CONTENTS

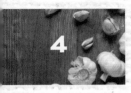
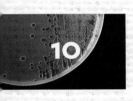
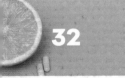
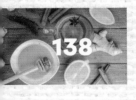

Introduction

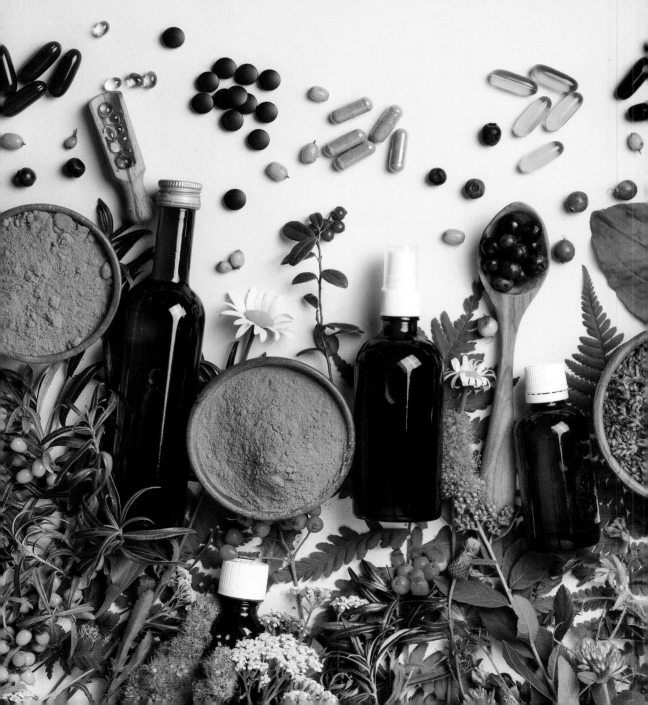

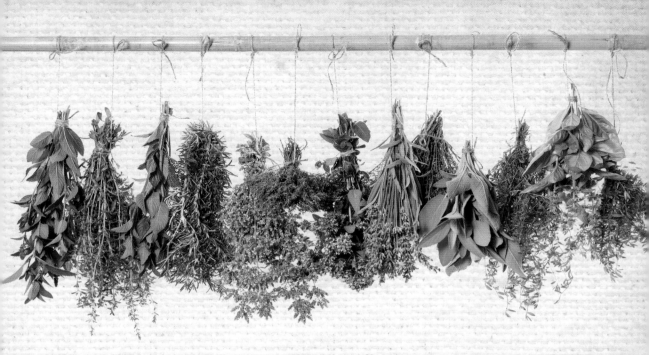

It is said that the era of modern antibiotics began in 1928, with Sir Alexander Fleming's discovery of penicillin. That era is not over, but right now its future looks grim. The rapid emergence of resistant bacteria is happening on a worldwide scale. The old antibiotics are less and less effective and few new ones are in development. While we may reasonably hope for eventual scientific breakthroughs to combat pathogens in the future, what do we do right now?

The obvious first answer is—stay healthy. By keeping our bodies illness-free, we eliminate the need for hospital visits and the overuse of antibiotics. That's where *Natural Antibiotics* can help. In this book, you'll discover natural, traditional sources for maintaining health and warding off illness. In-depth profiles on healing plants, from allspice to yarrow, can be found in chapter 3.

Natural cures for common ailments like colds and skin conditions can be found in chapter 4. Throughout, you'll find useful facts, notes on traditional uses, healing combinations and recipes, teas, blends, and salves, all of which you can make at home. These are the plants and preparations that have proven their worth in times past. There's no reason not to use them to help our bodies heal and be healthy now.

Stay well!

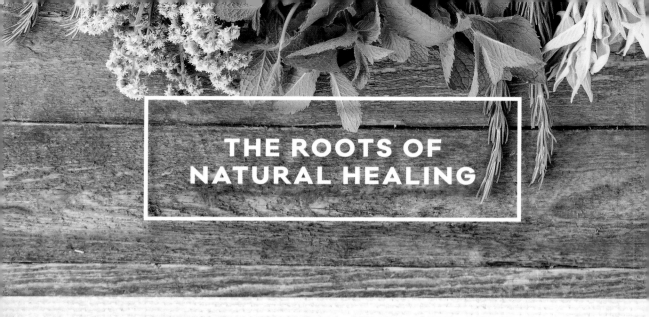

THE ROOTS OF NATURAL HEALING

The practice of healing with medicinal plants, fungi, and other natural substances is as old as the human species itself. The archaeological record is rich with evidence of herbs, roots, flowers, and seeds used to cure common ailments, infections, and disease. And based on recent research, we know that even our close relative, *Homo neanderthalensis*, was self-medicating 50,000 years ago. The remains of poplar (a natural source of aspirin), yarrow, chamomile, and even the *penicillium* fungus (from which we derive penicillin) have all been found in the dental remains of European Neanderthals.

The 1991 discovery of a 5,300-year-old frozen corpse in the Alps revealed that Ötzi the Iceman was treating his whipworm infestation with birch polypore (*Piptoporus betulinus*)—a potent natural antimicrobial. In Neolithic burial sites in Iran, medicinal plants like mint, horsetail, and nettle have been found carefully placed next to human remains. And the wine jars from ancient Egyptian tombs tell us that this culture developed sophisticated herbal concoctions and knew that alcohol was an excellent base to dissolve and administer them. Jar residue indicates the Egyptians may have used tree resins from pine and terebinth, and herbs like coriander, mint, rosemary, sage, savory, and thyme.

Whenever an ancient civilization has left behind written records, we invariably get a glimpse into how it diagnosed and treated illnesses. Sumerian clay tablets from 5,000 years ago reveal precise medical recipes that employed hundreds of plants. The Egyptian Ebers Papyrus, which is at least 3,500 years old, contains plant-based remedies that seem strikingly modern. But we also find that these ancient people knew a few things we have had to rediscover. A case in point is the use of pomegranate to treat parasitic worm infestations. Modern science has confirmed that the high tannin content of the pomegranate will actually paralyze the worms! What we see repeatedly in these ancient records is a deep and ingenious familiarity with nature's most powerful healing substances.

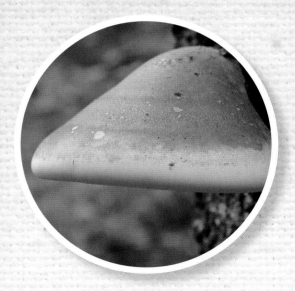

The birch polypore is a natural immune system booster and effective antiparasitic—a fact we now know Bronze Age Europeans took advantage of. Recent research has provided evidence that it is also anti-inflammatory, anticancer, neuroprotective, and immunomodulatory.

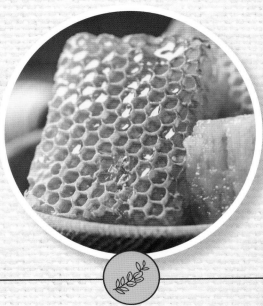

The Ebers Papyrus

This ancient medical compendium contains a large list of prescriptions using natural substances still familiar to us and often still used for the same purposes.
Among them:
- Aloe vera to alleviate burns and other skin conditions
- Caraway for digestion
- Castor oil as a laxative
- Honey for treating wounds
- Licorice for respiratory problems
- Onion to prevent the common cold

The Ebers Papyrus specified the use of honey for wound treatment. Human use of honey as a dressing for skin injuries is probably much older than recorded history. Research confirms that natural honey provides broad-spectrum protection against pathogenic bacteria, oral bacteria, and food spoilage bacteria.

Archaeological records indicate that humans have been using the castor plant for at least 7,000 years—possibly as both a poison and medicinally.

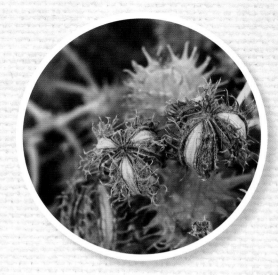

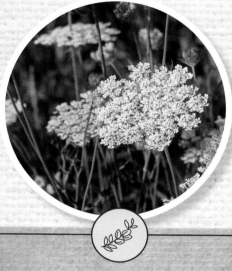

Caraway seeds have been found in ancient tombs, indicating the plant was held in high regard at least 5,000 years ago. Even earlier fossilized caraway seeds have been found at Neolithic and Mesolithic archaeological sites, some of which date back 8,000 years. For this reason, it is sometimes called Europe's oldest condiment. Written documents of its use in folk medicine—especially as a digestive aid—practically go back to the invention of writing.

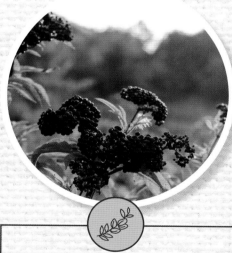

Archaeological excavations of Neolithic campsites across Europe have revealed the remains of the powerful antiviral elderberry.

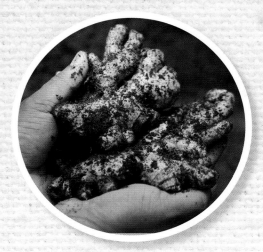

How long have humans been using ginger as a health tonic? Usage in India and China dates back at least 5,000 years.

The hardy oregano plant is another natural antibiotic with a history of use going back thousands of years. Ancient Egyptians, Babylonians, and Greeks all used oregano for respiratory illnesses, infections, and many other ailments.

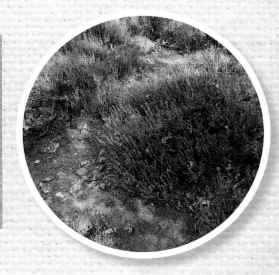

Modern medicine's development of antibiotics is one of its greatest achievements. But as overuse of common antibiotics leads to increasing resistance in microorganisms and the emergence of superbugs, older, time-proven, natural remedies have become relevant alternatives. As naturally occurring substances, they may not be standardized or as targeted as modern antimicrobial therapy, but they are still a viable means to heal and maintain health. And it's not an either/or situation—we are free to use both. Familiarizing ourselves with these gentle, body-friendly sources can only lead to good things—fewer illnesses, fewer trips to the doctor, less pharmaceutical use, and a more productive life.

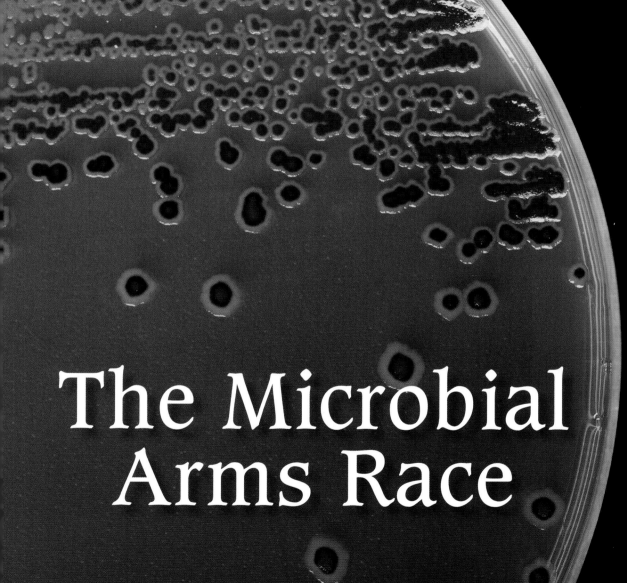

The Microbial
Arms Race

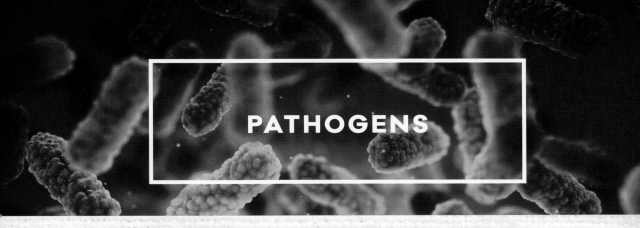

PATHOGENS

Pathogens, simply put, are agents that can cause disease. Sometimes called germs or infectious agents, pathogens are typically microorganisms such as bacteria, fungi, or viruses. Some pathogens, like the hepatitis C virus, are deadly or can produce lifelong effects in humans. Others—rhinoviruses (the common cold), for example—are far more common and less frightening.

Bacterial Pathogens

Many bacteria either have no effect on humans or are actually helpful to the human body. Thousands of species of bacteria, for instance, exist in the human digestive system and serve important roles in the processing of food. Bacterial pathogens are bacteria that cause disease, and the number of species of those is much smaller—several hundred, perhaps. Each species of such bacteria can cause specific symptoms in people who become infected, particularly those with compromised immune systems. Many times, however, there are no symptoms at all.

The symptoms, of course, can be of great help in diagnosing the bacterial pathogen at work. Bacterial pneumonia, for example, is an infection of the lungs. There are many types of bacterial skin infections that affect cut/scraped areas of the skin. Bacterial meningitis is an inflammation of the membranes protecting the brain and spinal cord. Urinary tract infections are caused primarily by bacteria. There are many others.

Antibiotics are typically used to treat such diseases. However, a 2013 CDCP report outlining changes in antibiotic resistance called such resistance "one of the biggest public health challenges of our time." The report noted that at least two million people contract an antibiotic-resistant infection and more than 23,000 people die from such infections every year in the United States. More than 1,000 of those deaths were related to bacterial pathogens commonly transmitted through food. Salmonella was the biggest culprit for both number of hospitalizations and deaths.

The ability of bacteria to develop resistance to antibiotics is receiving a great amount of study, as medical science works diligently to develop new solutions for treatment. Increasing numbers of multidrug resistant (MDR) and extremely drug-resistant (XDR) bacterial pathogens continue to emerge. The O'Neill report, released in 2016 in the United Kingdom, estimated that by 2050 about 10 million people per year would be dying from antibiotic-resistant infections.

The World Health Organization, in 2017, released a global priority pathogens list of antibiotic-resistant bacteria to help prioritize the research and development of new antibiotic treatments. The WHO list included 12 bacteria or bacterial families divided into three categories: critical, high and medium. The list:

Critical: *Acinetobacter baumannii* (carbapenem-resistant); *Pseudomonas aeruginosa* (carbapenem-resistant); and *Enterobacteriaceae*, including *Klebsiella pneumonia*, *Escherichia coli*, *Enterobacter species*, *Serratia* species, *Proteus* species, *Providencia* species and *Morganella* species (carbapenem-resistant, third-generation cephalosporin-resistant).

High: *Enterococcus faecium* (vancomycin-resistant); *Staphylococcus aureus* (methicillin-resistant, vancomycin intermediate and resistant); *Helicobacter pylori* (clarithromycin-resistant); *Campylobacter* (fluoroquinolone-resistant); *Salmonella* species (fluoroquinolone-resistant); and *Neisseria gonorrhoeae* (third-generation cephalosporin-resistant, fluoroquinolone-resistant).

Medium: *Streptococcus pneumoniae* (penicillin-non-susceptible); *Haemophilus influenzae* (ampicillin-resistant); and *Shigella species* (fluoroquinolone-resistant).

One deadly pathogenic bacteria not included in the WHO report because it has long been established as a critical global priority is *Mycobacteria*, including *Mycobacterium tuberculosis*. Tuberculosis, historically called consumption, is an ancient disease thought to infect some 25 percent of the world population.

Particularly prevalent in sub-Saharan Africa, tuberculosis can infect many parts of the body but is particularly damaging to the lungs. Vaccination and early detection are crucial, as treating the disease with multiple rounds of antibiotics has become a challenge due to the growing antibiotic resistance of some bacteria. While the number of new cases of tuberculosis has been on the decline since 2000, its deadly nature in developing countries remains a critical problem.

The CDC also released a threats report in 2013 that included several bacterial pathogens among the "urgent" and "serious" threats to human beings due to antibiotic resistance. Among the most urgent were *C. difficile*, which can cause life-threatening diarrhea and inflammation of the colon; Nightmare bacteria, including a family of germs called *Enterobacteriaceae* that are resistant to almost all antibiotics; and *N. gonorrhoeae*, which causes the STD gonorrhea that has grown to develop resistance to the antibiotics that have been prescribed to fight it.

Whether to combat tuberculosis or other MDR or XDR bacterial pathogens, scientists agree that there is an urgent need to develop new antibiotic compounds. This effort can take a number of different approaches. Among the possibilities: designing new antibiotic derivatives, with improved properties, from an already known family of antibiotics; finding novel chemical structures to fight existing bacteria; or exploring alternative therapeutics (this can be difficult due to regulatory restrictions).

Fungal Pathogens

Millions of different fungal species can be found on earth, but only about 300 are known to cause human illness. Some can do serious damage. Candida is one such pathogen. There are more than 20 species of these yeasts that can cause human infection, the most common being *Candida albicans*. The CDC listed candida among its "serious" antibiotic-resistant threats in a 2013 report, attributing more than 200 annual deaths to this fungal pathogen. *Candida auris*—an emerging, multidrug-resistant fungus that has been considered a serious global health threat—is gaining a great deal of scientific attention.

Ringworm: A circular rash typically shaped like a ring, this is a common skin infection that often causes redness and itchiness. The fungi that causes this infection can live on the skin, or pretty much any household items or surfaces.

Aspergillosis: The common *Aspergillus* mold lives both indoors and outdoors. Most people who breathe it, even on an everyday basis, do so without getting sick. But for people with weakened immune systems, Aspergillosis can result in allergic reactions and lung infections.

Cryptococcus: Though the majority of this species live in the soil and do not cause harm to humans, they sometimes trigger a form of meningitis in those who have HIV or AIDS. There are also types that are capable of causing disease in people whose immune systems are not compromised.

Fungal nail infections: Discoloring of the fingernails or toenails can be caused by any number of fungi (yeasts or molds). Some people can also develop a fungal skin infection on the foot, more commonly known as "athlete's foot." Antifungal creams or pills can be used to combat these infections, but treatment usually takes a long time.

Histoplasmosis: Common in soil that contains a large quantity of bird or bat droppings, the *Histoplasma* fungus is prevalent in the Ohio and Mississippi River valleys in the United States. Most people who breathe in these spores do not become sick, but fever, coughing and fatigue are possible for some.

Pneumocystis pneumonia (PCP): Once classified as a protozoan, *Pneumocystis jirovecii* is now considered a fungus. Most people who get PCP from it are those whose immune systems are weakened by the likes of HIV or AIDS. Still, PCP is considered a substantial public health problem.

Stachybotrys chartarum: Also known as black mold, this species can cause problems for those living in wet or damp homes. Typical symptoms include respiratory issues and severe, lingering headaches.

Blastomycosis: Breathing in a fungus called *Blastomyces* can cause this infection, whose symptoms can resemble those of the flu. The fungus is most prominent in the U.S. and Canada around the Ohio and Mississippi River valley regions, typically in moist soil or decomposing wood and leaves.

Viral Pathogens

British biologist Sir Peter Brian Medawar once called a virus "a piece of bad news wrapped in a protein coat." Regardless of their makeup, pathogenic viruses are bad news, as they cause some of the most dangerous diseases known. Cell death leading to tissue damage accounts for the pathology of many human viral diseases. Infections can be chronic, grow worse over time, or a virus can even enter a latent state while remaining capable of reactivation.

Hepatitis viruses: Hepatitis is a generic term referring to inflammation of the liver, but more than half of all cases of acute hepatitis in the United States are viral. Viral hepatitis is commonly caused by one of three viruses: hepatitis A (HAV), hepatitis B (HBV) and hepatitis C (HCV). Many RNA and DNA viruses target the liver, and inhibit its ability to regulate metabolism and blood composition.

Arboviruses: Arboviruses are groups of viruses transmitted by mosquitoes, fleas, ticks and other invertebrates—insects known as arthropods. They include flaviviruses, alphaviruses, and bunya viruses. Typically, an infection will progress to symptoms that can last up to two weeks but also lifelong immunity from the infection. Examples of such diseases include Yellow fever, Dengue fever, West Nile fever, and tick-borne encephalitis.

Herpesviruses: There are more than 100 known herpesviruses, but just eight impact only humans. They are the herpes simplex virus types 1 and 2, varicella-zoster virus, cytomegalovirus, Epstein-Barr virus, human herpesvirus 6 (variants A and B), human herpesvirus 7, and Kaposi's sarcoma virus or human herpesvirus 8. Almost every human is infected with one or more of these viruses, which range from cold sores and chicken pox to latent infections that can contribute to cancer.

Polyomaviruses: Small, nonenveloped DNA viruses that are widespread throughout nature, these viruses remain latent after primary infection in human hosts with competent immune systems. In almost all cases, humans become ill after contact with these viruses only if their immune systems are already compromised.

Respiratory viruses: The respiratory system is so intricate and vital, it's imperative that we account for the numerous viruses that make regular attacks on it. Respiratory viruses are among the most common causes of illness in humans. Influenza viruses, respiratory syncytial virus (RSV), parainfluenza viruses, and respiratory adenoviruses are among the attackers. Several of these viral pathogens cause similar symptoms, compromising the upper respiratory tract and producing fever, chills, headaches, body aches, general weakness, and breathing difficulty, to list some. They can also cause complications like tonsillitis, laryngitis, bronchitis, and pneumonia. Influenza viruses are highly contagious, can be deadly and can lead to epidemics. That's why every year flu vaccines are developed to combat the ever-changing viruses.

Papillomaviruses: Papillomaviruses are a family of small viruses that infect virtually all mammals. PVs cause infections without triggering the immune system, which can make them particularly harmful. Their presentations can range from small warts on the skin to certain kinds of cancer (cervical and anal cancer among them).

Parvoviruses: Parvoviruses are small, single-stranded DNA genomes that can cause viral infections in humans and animals. One of the most common among humans is Parvovirus B19, which can cause "fifth disease" in children (causing a red-cheeked appearance).

Rhabdoviruses: The name of these viruses comes from the Greek "rhabdos," meaning "rod," which describes the shape of the viral particles. The most well known of these is the rabies virus, which frequently stems from animal bites and causes acute infection of the central nervous system—potentially leading to death if it is left untreated.

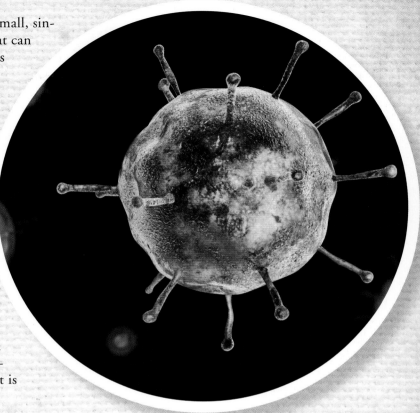

Retroviruses: Retroviruses operate a little differently than most viruses. Instead of its genes being encoded in DNA, retrovirus genes are encoded in RNA. This requires an additional step for infection to take place, as the retrovirus genome needs to be reversed transcribed into one's DNA. This reversal to the typical gene copying process resulted in the name "retro." HIV is an example of a retrovirus affecting humans. Another is the human T-cell lymphotropic virus 1 (HTLV-1), which is associated with certain T-cell leukemias and lymphomas.

During peak flu season in the United States, anywhere between 5 and 20% of the population will come down with the illness. During the 2017–2018 season, the Centers for Disease Control and Prevention estimated that nearly 49 million people suffered a flu episode.

Parasitical Pathogens

A parasite is an organism that lives inside a host organism and gains sustenance from its host. The parasite is physiologically dependent on its host for survival. Parasites can cause disease in humans and animals. The three main types that cause human infections are protozoa, helminths and ectoparasites. Here, we will take a look at each of the three.

Protozoa are microscopic, single-cell organisms that can be parasitic but can also live freely outside a host. Because they can multiply rapidly in humans, their ability to survive, thrive, and cause serious infections despite their single-cell nature is great. Protozoa living in the human intestine are typically transferred through a fecal/oral path (contaminated food or water, for example), while those living in the blood can be transferred via insect (i.e., mosquito) bites.

There are several diseases related to protozoa infections, the most well-known and deadly of which is malaria. According to the Centers for Disease Control and Prevention (CDC), malaria kills more than 600,000 people every year—mostly children in sub-Saharan Africa. Mosquito bites are responsible for more than half of malaria cases around the world. Other protozoan diseases include toxoplasmosis and Chagas disease.

Helminths, unlike protozoa, are multi-cell organisms that can typically be seen with the naked eye and, in their adult form, cannot multiply inside humans. The word derives from

Infected ticks transmit Lyme disease-causing bacteria via their saliva when they bite. A tick usually has to be attached to a host for 24 hours before this occurs, but shorter transmission times have been recorded.

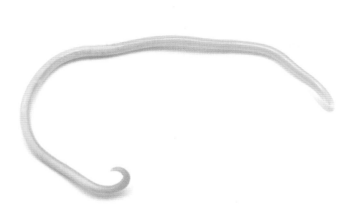

the Greek for "worms." Like protozoa, they can live inside a host or on their own. Helminth infestations can compromise nutritional status, affect cognitive process, induce tissue reactions and cause intestinal obstruction or rectal prolapse. They are particularly common among children.

There are three main groups that operate as parasites within humans and can cause disease—flatworms (such as tapeworms), thorny-headed worms (these generally live in the gastrointestinal tract), and roundworms (these can do damage within several internal organs).

Close to one billion people worldwide are thought to be infected with the common roundworm, according to the Royal Pharmaceutical Society.

Ectoparasites can typically include insects like mosquitoes, because they are reliant on blood from a human for their survival. For the study of parasitical pathogens, however, the term refers to organisms like ticks, fleas, mites and lice that can attach to the skin or burrow into it. Lyme disease, scabies, myiasis, and many skin disorders are among the many infections that can be attributed to ectoparasites.

Deer ticks are the leading transmitter of Lyme disease, a multisystem inflammatory disease that's now considered the most common arthropod-borne illness in the United States. Common in the Northeast and Midwest due to its carrier, it is typical of an ectoparasitic pathogen in that early detection and antibiotic treatment lead to a very high success rate.

The Advantage of Natural Antibiotics

The term *natural antibiotic* is used in the popular sense in this book. Originally, antibiotics referred to substances produced by microorganisms that inhibited the growth of other microorganisms. As synthetic antibiotics came into use, the term came to refer to these pharmaceutical products. Synthetic antibiotics typically target bacteria—not viruses, fungi, or protozoan pathogens. But the term has since gained wide public recognition as any kind of pharmaceutical agent used to kill "germs." This book is similarly broad in its use of the term. The word *natural* is used to clearly differentiate from standard pharmaceutical antibiotics. Strictly speaking, the natural substances we use to combat pathogens harmful to humans would be better termed *antimicrobials*. The term is broader in scope and indicates the substance is active against all classes of microorganisms.

One of the great advantages of natural antibiotics is that the bioactive properties of these substances are *broad spectrum*. Standard pharmaceutical antibiotics are typically *narrow spectrum*—only effective against one or a few germs. Few pharmaceutical antibiotics will be effective against protozoans. Even fewer will have an effect on fungi. And none work against viruses. Not so with the antimicrobials found in nature. These agents have robust properties that allow them to be effective in multiple ways and on multiple fronts.

Natural antibiotics, simply by being present in the body, may create a toxic environment for germs. This action is twofold: as a *bactericide* (capable of killing bacteria outright), substances in natural antibiotics initiate dissolution of germs via enzymatic breakdown. Natural antibiotics can also create a *bacteriostatic effect*, meaning that they inhibit the growth or reproduction of bacteria. Germs stop multiplying because they are under attack. They defend themselves by thickening their membranes. This compromises their ability to communicate with their environment and inhibits cellular multiplication.

Natural antibiotics can create a hostile environment for fungi and protozoans as well. This is something pharmaceutical antibiotics have yet to do on a significant level. Essentially, natural antibiotics optimize the cellular terrain for human health, and make the terrain hostile for germs. Simultaneously, natural antibiotics help to eliminate toxins and correct deficiencies in the organism. This cleansing eliminates the metabolic waste that some germs feed on. Natural antibiotics can also stimulate the physiological functions that make a body less susceptible to infection—they kick the body's immune responses into high gear.

When compared to pharmaceutical antibiotics, natural antibiotics have a number of spectacular advantages, but in a time of superbugs and resistant bacteria, one may trump all others: in most cases, *germs do not develop a resistance to them.* There are multiple reasons for this, but one simply comes down to molecular complexity. **Biologically active molecules in natural antibiotics are vastly more complex and numerous than the single-molecule approach of synthetic antibiotics**. Germs cannot develop all the enzymes and defensive strategies necessary to deal with this complexity. Something else to consider: natural antibiotics are gentle on the body. They don't cause dehydration, bloating, diarrhea, or destroy native gut flora. A lack of side effects means the body can focus on healing itself.

Proof in the Pudding

Cultures across the world have learned that certain plants have medicinal qualities. They have learned this through direct experience. The fact that the medical establishment, particularly in the United States, tends to disregard the efficacy of natural antibiotics does not invalidate them. As we learned above, natural antibiotics are broad spectrum in their effects. In most cases, we need not worry about how long we use them, diminishing efficacy, toxic byproducts, or other unpleasant side effects. For this reason, we can expect a holistic healing experience when we use them. Natural antibiotics are not only *against* pathogens, they are also *for* health.

Key Terms

Antimicrobial
Inhibits the growth of a variety of microorganisms (including bacteria, fungi, protozoa, and viruses).

Antibacterial
Specifically targets bacteria.

Antifungal
Specifically targets fungi.

Antiviral
Specifically targets viruses.

Antiparasitic
Specifically targets parasites.

Words ending with –cide
Indicates the substance kills pathogens in that category (e.g., a fungicide kills fungi).

Antiseptic
An antimicrobial substance that is applied to living tissue to prevent, treat, or reduce infection.

Disinfectant
An antimicrobial substance that is applied to non-living surfaces like countertops, sinks, and equipment.

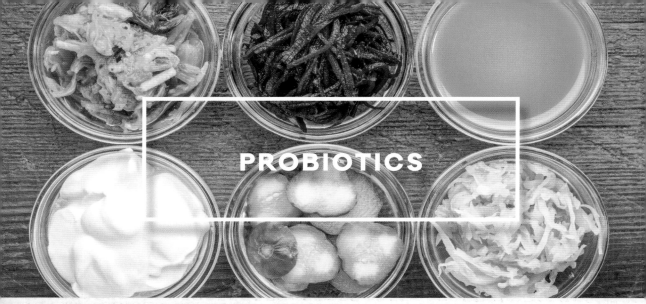

PROBIOTICS

The human body is loaded with bacteria. Trillions of microorganisms live within our bodies, with bacterial cells often outnumbering human cells. While this might sound like a problematic mix, keep in mind that the vast majority of the bacteria in the human body are either harmless or, in fact, helpful. Most of the time, these trillions of microorganisms live harmoniously with their human hosts, contributing to many vital functions essential to survival.

According to the U.S. Health and Human Services, nearly every human being carries pathogens. Yet in healthy people these pathogens do not lead to disease. Bacteria that resides in the gut can play a key role in keeping pathogens from causing illness. They also contribute to better immune function, digestion, and in preventing those pathogens from doing harm.

However, scientists and medical professionals also know that imbalances among the cells and bacteria that live in the human body can contribute to illnesses and disorders. The term probiotic comes from the Latin *pro* (for) and *biota* (life). Probiotics are live, "good" bacteria (or yeasts, in some instances) that are the same or similar to bacteria that already exist in the human body. Though proof is hard to come by, there is a good deal of evidence that probiotics may be helpful in keeping the ecosystem of the human body—particularly the digestive system—balanced and healthy.

Probiotics can be taken in both food and supplement form.

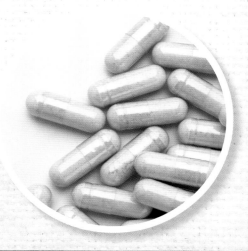

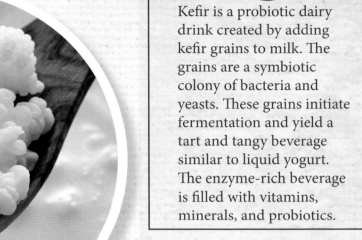

Kefir is a probiotic dairy drink created by adding kefir grains to milk. The grains are a symbiotic colony of bacteria and yeasts. These grains initiate fermentation and yield a tart and tangy beverage similar to liquid yogurt. The enzyme-rich beverage is filled with vitamins, minerals, and probiotics.

Fermentation

While probiotics seem, to most, rather new and lightly studied in the world of science, the concepts actually date back thousands of years. Fermentation is a process by which sugars and starches in food break down and turn into an alcohol or acid. Fermentation can be traced back to ancient times. Fermented products were probably found or discovered, rather than created. Legend holds that yogurt, considered a natural probiotic, derived from a fermentation process within the animal skin bags used to transport milk and water in Middle Asia and the Middle East, places where temperatures are high and humidity low.

Elie Metchnikoff, a Nobel laureate, is often called the "father of probiotics" or "father of natural immunity" for his work in the field about 150 years ago. In the late 1800s, this ground-breaking Russian scientist inoculated himself with a relapsing fever to learn if it was transmissible by blood. The effects on him were severe, as fever frequently led to death in those days, but he survived and went on to evangelize the notion that the flora of the human intestine could be bolstered with the ingestion of fermented milk. It would become the debut of "modern" probiotics.

There has been a great deal of study over the past few decades about probiotics. There is now clinical evidence that probiotics can be helpful, particularly in treating disorders of the stomach and digestive system. Further study is ongoing and necessary, and a big reason why trial-and-error is still a common approach to probiotic treatment and supplementation.

Types of Probiotics

There are many types of bacteria classified as probiotics, but most of them fall into two large categories—*lactobacillus* and *bifidobacterium*.

Lactobacillus is the type found in yogurt, cheese, sauerkraut, pickles, beer, cider, and other fermented foods, along with many dietary supplements. It has been used to help treat and prevent diarrhea, including rotaviral diarrhea in children, traveler's diarrhea, and other infectious types of diarrhea. It has also been used to prevent and treat diarrhea linked to the use of antibiotics.

Lactobacillus has also been used for several other common issues, including the inability to digest the lactose in milk. Some have used it for IBS (irritable bowel syndrome), colic in babies, colon inflammation, urinary tract infections, vaginal yeast infections, and even the common cold and high cholesterol. Along with these conditions or illnesses, skin disorders such as fever blisters, canker sores, and acne have been combatted with lactobacillus. While some swear by its effectiveness, not enough evidence exists to draw firm conclusions.

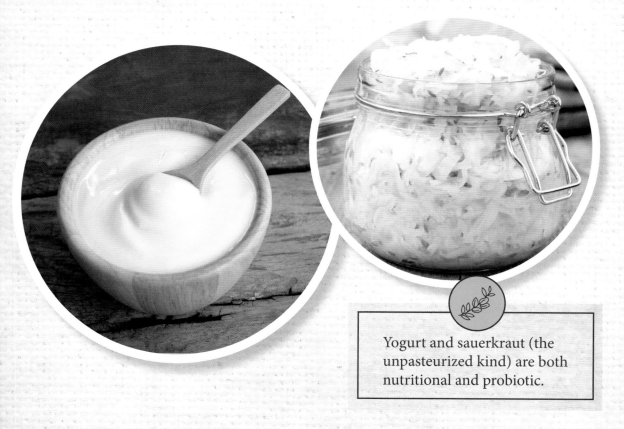

Yogurt and sauerkraut (the unpasteurized kind) are both nutritional and probiotic.

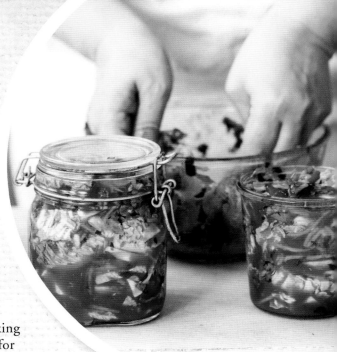

Bifidobacterium is generally found in the intestines, but the group of bacteria can also be grown outside the body and then taken orally as a probiotic. These bacteria are frequently used to treat and prevent some of the same conditions as lactobacillus— the common cold or flu, IBS and diarrhea among them.

Bifidobacteria belong to the lactic acid bacteria group. When diseases spring up in the human body and destroy some of the "good" bacteria that typically keep the body functioning in good health, these bacteria can be introduced to help "even up" the battle. According to WebMD, research indicates that taking bifidobacteria may increase bowel movements for those with constipation by 2–4 per week.

In addition to the conditions mentioned above, bifidobacteria have been used to combat ulcerative colitis. Numerous other conditions and illnesses have been treated with bifidobacteria, but there is not enough evidence to vouch for their effectiveness against eczema, diabetes, arthritis, allergies and a variety of others.

One other grouping of probiotics that has received substantial study is known as *Saccharomyces boulardii*. This refers to a type of yeast found in many probiotics that has been correlated in some circles to effectiveness in fighting digestive system and diarrhea issues.

It should be noted that the U.S. Food and Drug Administration (FDA) has not approved any probiotic for the prevention or treatment of any health issue, according to the U.S. Department of Health and Human Services. Probiotic supplements, therefore, do not have FDA signoff and it's a good idea to get a physician's opinion before beginning a probiotic treatment plan.

Kimchi is a Korean fermented cabbage preparation typically including garlic, scallions, ginger, and chili powder. The vegetables are fermented with a number of bacteria, of which lactic acid bacteria are dominant. The result is a pungent, spicy side dish with lots of nutrients, probiotics, and fiber.

Science and Probiotics

Although the FDA does not regulate the probiotic supplement industry, science does have plenty to say about these "good" bacteria. Among healthy individuals, there have been very minimal side effects—usually mild digestive system issues. That's probably because there are so many microorganisms within the human body, the addition of "good" bacteria is rarely able to disrupt the ecosystem in a negative way. For those with underlying medical problems or weakened immune systems, however, there is reason to tread cautiously with probiotics. There have been instances of severe effects such as infections.

Lactobacillus and bifidobacterium have undergone in-depth studies, while some of the other probiotics have not been subject to that kind of scrutiny. Thus, what might be considered safe with a certain probiotic might not be safe with a probiotic from a different class.

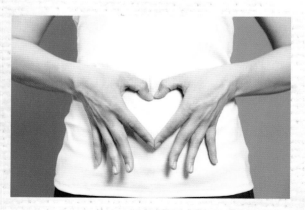

Additionally, because the FDA has not put its stamp of approval on probiotic supplements, shoppers should be cautious as to what's inside any bottle or container. Read the labels carefully, and always consult with a primary care physician.

The Gut

The term "gut flora" (or gut microbiota) refers to the complex—and, at times, delicate—balance of microorganisms in the human digestive tract. The largest number of bacteria and the greatest number of species live here. The composition changes over time, and the way the bacteria and cells interact with one another is critical to the ability of humans to digest food and maintain health.

Probiotics have been effective in digestive health, for reasons that might include these: maintaining a stable and desirable community of microorganisms; strengthening or stabilizing the barriers that keep undesirable bacteria out of the digestive tract; helping the community of microorganisms return to "normal" after a disturbance such as a disease or effects of antibiotic use; "bulking up the ecosystem" with good bacteria to battle the potentially harmful ones; or simulating the body's immune system.

Harvard Medical School took a look at two recent studies and determined that probiotics might reduce antibiotic-associated diarrhea by 60 percent when compared with a placebo. The school also cited several other studies in suggesting that certain probiotics might help maintain remission of ulcerative colitis and prevent relapse of Crohn's disease.

Though Harvard noted that the "jury is still out" when it comes to specific recommendations for probiotic treatment of certain digestive tract problems (and other conditions), the renowned medical school continues to pursue advances when it comes to probiotics and the gut.

Vaginal Health

The same can be said for the potential probiotic benefits to vaginal health. Like the digestive tract, the vagina is a delicately balanced ecosystem of microorganisms that makes it susceptible to its own unique infections and conditions. The lactobacilli strains that dominate that system normally do an effective job keeping harmful bacteria from causing issues in healthy women.

A number of things, however, can throw off the fine balance. Among them: spermicides, antibiotics, and birth control pills. Probiotics that help restore the body's balance may be effective in fighting or preventing issues like yeast infections, urinary tract infections (UTIs) and bacterial vaginosis, among others. Studies are being pursued every day to uncover other potential benefits to vaginal and reproductive health.

Old folklore holds that yogurt, either eaten (most commonly) or inserted into the vagina (less commonly), can help conquer yeast infections. Science has little to say about this idea, which unfortunately keeps it in the folklore category. Vaginosis calls for more conventional treatment due to the risk of pelvic inflammatory disease and possible pregnancy complications. As with other probiotic treatments, their use to battle UTIs is being widely studied, and more study is necessary.

Probiotics and Weight Loss

Another area where probiotics are undergoing extensive study is the weight loss realm. Given many people's intense desire to lose weight as quickly and easily as possible, it's no surprise that probiotic supplement companies are quick to tout their products as a way to fast-track a slimmer waist, much like the unproven methods of injecting pregnancy hormones or taking ephedrine supplements have been touted in the past.

With probiotics, however, there seems to be a good deal of promise. One 2013 study published in the U.S. National Library of Medicine found that in 210 people with obesity characterized by excess belly fat, daily ingestion of the probiotic *lactobacillus gasseri* (considered the leading probiotic helper in this category) led to an 8.5-percent reduction in that fat over a 12-week period. Participants began regaining the fat within four weeks of when they stopped supplementing.

Some have hypothesized that overweight and obese patients tend to have more bad bacteria in their gut than those who are lean, and that taking probiotic supplements can help achieve a better gut flora balance leading to weight loss. Complicating the hypothesis, though, is the fact that science cannot currently tell whether gut bacteria occurred organically or as a result of eating and exercise habits.

In other words, good diet and proper exercise are the staples of maintaining healthy weight. "We're still very early in our understanding of our gut biome and how it affects weight," Dr. Scott Kahan, director of the National Center for Weight and Wellness, told *Men's Health*.

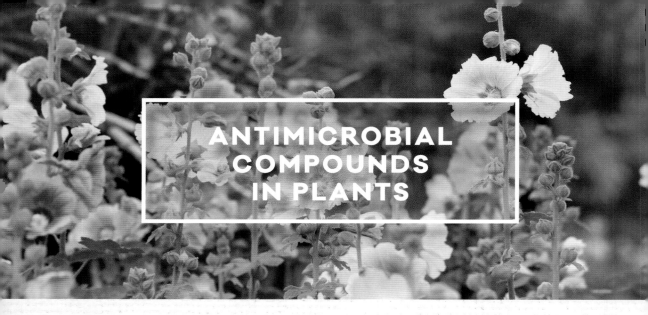

ANTIMICROBIAL COMPOUNDS IN PLANTS

The use of plants for healing and the prevention of illnesses appears to be the oldest form of medicine in the world. There is evidence that as long as 60,000 years ago, Neanderthals living in what is now Iraq used hollyhock (above) for such purposes. That flowering plant remains in use as a healer in many parts of the world today. In the late 5th century BC, Hippocrates wrote about hundreds of medicinal plants and their uses. To this day, doctors commit to the Hippocratic oath—named in his honor—as the standard of their profession.

Plant oils and extracts have been used to battle illnesses and in food preservation for thousands of years. In the famous bible story, frankincense and myrrh were among the first gifts brought to the newborn baby Jesus. They were not random offerings. These compounds are known to have antiseptic properties used in healing and wellness, and they show up elsewhere in the bible, too.

Chinese medicine incorporates more than 3,000 years of history in using a natural, holistic approach to healing. *The Imperial* *Grace Formulary* of the Tai Ping Era (AD 985) documents 16,834 herbal entities used to preserve or treat illnesses. In fact, Chinese herbal medicine has served as a foundation for American and British medicine in many ways over many years.

On American soil, one need look no further than Native Americans to witness the use of herbal remedies. Sage was used to treat a variety of stomach, kidney, liver and skin problems. American ginseng was thought to be one of the best options to combat the common cold. And dogwood was used by many tribes to battle flu and fever symptoms.

Not surprisingly, modern science has devoted considerable time to affirming and debunking some of the plant-based treatments that have been used for thousands and thousands of years. To the surprise of few, there is evidence to support the notion that practitioners of these natural remedies were—in many cases—onto something.

Secondary Metabolites

Secondary metabolites are organic compounds which are not directly involved in the growth or survival of the organism but which may handle other functions such as protection, species interaction, or competition. Antimicrobial peptides (pAMPs), first discovered in 1942, are produced by bacteria, animals, and plants to serve as natural defense compounds against disease-causing pathogens. Research shows that pAMPs are a key component of plants' defense against pathogens.

Thionins. The first pAMPs to be discovered in the mid-20th century, thionins are toxic to yeast, fungi, and bacteria. It is thought that the way they bind themselves to cell membranes in large numbers can cause damage to pathogens. Viscotoxin, found in European mistletoe, is one of the most well-known thionins. There is evidence of its effectiveness against tumor cells, causing membrane damage that leads to destabilization and lipid bi-layer disruption.

Plant Defensins. Plant defensins, which have been derived from tubers, leaves, pods, seeds, and flowers, are capable of inhibiting bacteria and fungi. Because they do so with no lethal effect against plant or animal cells, they have been of particular interest as preservative agents for food—able to help preserve while doing no damage.

Lipid Transfer Proteins. Isolated from barley, maize, spinach, broccoli, and radish, among others, LTPs have not undergone as much study as other pAMPs but have demonstrated an important role in pathogen defense. Their ability to inhibit microbial growth is particularly promising. Very effective against fungi but also against certain types of bacteria, LTPs were once thought to be involved in the transfer of lipids—hence the name.

Myrosinase-binding Proteins. MBPs are involved in plant development and defense, primarily against fungi, bacteria, and insects. They act in microbial membranes.

Hevein- and Knottin-like Peptides. Found in seeds and other plant tissues, HTPs were first isolated from rubber latex. They inhibit fungi and bacteria and are thus considered a promising food preservative.

Snakins. Isolated from potatoes, Snakins are antimicrobials that show activity against fungi and bacteria. They are a relatively new antimicrobial peptide and continue to be studied for both their medical potential and as a natural preservative.

Cyclotides. Kalata B1, the first cyclotide identified, works against nematodes and insects, as well as showing inhibition of human immunodeficiency virus (HIV). Other cyclotides have showed activity against animal cells and *E. coli*. Divided into two subfamilies—Mobius and bracelet—cyclotides show great potential to serve as novel antibiotics in controlling infectious diseases.

Peptides from Hydrolysates. Beans are hugely popular in many countries around the world, and hydrolysates from leguminous plants are making a big impact against bacteria. One study indicated that the hydrolysates of rapeseed protein inhibited the protease activity of human immunodeficiency virus (HIV) that was expressed in *E. coli* cells.

Phytochemicals

In addition to secondary metabolites, phytochemicals found in plants also work as important antimicrobial agents. These naturally occurring chemicals provide plants with odor, color, and flavor. More importantly for humans, ingesting these phytochemicals can impact the chemical processes inside our bodies for the better. According to the American Institute for Cancer Research, laboratory studies have shown that phytochemicals have the potential to:

• Stimulate the immune system
• Block substances we eat, drink, and breathe from becoming carcinogens
• Reduce the kind of inflammation that makes cancer growth more likely
• Prevent DNA damage and help with DNA repair
• Reduce the kind of oxidative damage to cells that can spark cancer
• Slow the growth rate of cancer cells
• Trigger damaged cells to commit suicide before they can reproduce

Doctors recommend a diet high in a variety of vegetables, fruits, whole grains and beans, and note that brightly colored and strong flavored fruits and vegetables tend to be the best sources of phytochemicals. Thousands of phytochemicals have been identified. They can be divided into categories like simple phenolic compounds, flavonoids, quinones, tannins, and coumarins. The most important phytochemicals, when it comes to food preservation, are essential oils. Their preservation properties were realized in ancient times, while many of the others are much more recent discoveries. Following is a glance at some of the various types of phytochemicals and their potential benefits.

Carotenoids: These are found in red, orange, and green fruits and vegetables such as carrots, cooked tomatoes, leafy greens, sweet potatoes, winter squash, apricots, cantaloupe, oranges, and watermelon. They may work as antioxidants, improve immune response and potentially inhibit the growth of cancer cells.

Flavones, Flavonols, and Flavonoids: Apples, citrus fruits, onions, soybeans, and soy products (tofu, soy milk, edamame, and the like), coffee, and tea contain flavonoids such as anthocyanins and quercetin. They are thought to be effective in fighting a number of microorganisms due to their ability to bind to and inactivate proteins. These phytochemicals may improve immune response and the production of detoxifying enzymes in the body, and might also inhibit inflammation and the growth of tumors.

Indoles and Glucosinolates: Cruciferous vegetables such as broccoli, cabbage, collard greens, kale, cauliflower, and Brussels sprouts all contain these phytochemicals, which are thought to block carcinogens and spark their detoxification. There is also some evidence that they might help limit the production of hormones related to cancer.

Inositol: A known antioxidant, this can be found in bran from corn, oats, rice, rye, and wheat, along with nuts, soybeans, and soy products like edamame.

Polyphenols: Green tea, grapes, wine, berries, citrus fruits, apples, whole grains, and peanuts are among the sources of these phytochemicals.

They are thought to prevent inflammation and work as antioxidants, and cancer researchers are particularly interested in their potential in the prevention of the disease's formation.

Quinones: Much like flavones, flavonols, and flavonoids, quinones put their antimicrobial properties to use by binding inactive proteins. One of the biggest applications of quinones is in the production of hydrogen peroxide, with several billion kilograms produced each year.

Tannins and Coumarins: You might have heard about tannins in wine or coffee. They occur in fruit, nuts, and seeds, and exhibit antimicrobial characteristics against fungi, viruses, and bacteria, including—importantly—antibiotic-resistant strains. They have also been shown to be toxic to yeasts and some fungi. Coumarin is a vanilla-scented compound found naturally in plants that shows antioxidant and anti-inflammatory characteristics.

Essential Oils: As noted earlier, this is the big one when it comes to food preservation. These volatile compounds are aptly named *essential*. Also called terpenes, these oils have been demonstrated to hold anti-inflammatory, antiviral, and anticancer effects along with antioxidant properties. Cherries, citrus fruit peel, rosemary, thyme, tea tree, and mint are among the many producers of essential oils.

Planting the Future

So many compounds in foods readily available to most Americans have shown their potential mettle in defending against pathogens and disease. Spices such as garlic, clove, cinnamon, ginger, and black pepper can be added to that mix. Eating brightly colored fruits and vegetables has long been a credo of doctors advising their patients on wellness.

The list of ailments that may be impacted by natural, plant-based remedies reads like a who's-who of issues impacting global health. Cancer, cardiovascular disease, Type 2 diabetes, and neurodegeneration are among the diseases that might be greatly impacted by antimicrobial compounds found in common plants.

There are some risks to be aware of, and for this reason it's recommended that you consult with your physician before leaning into natural remedies as a solution. Though these remedies have been around for a while, science has limited data compared to its work in more conventional antibiotics. The long-range effects of large amounts of phytochemicals on health are not known. Their role as antioxidants is documented, but as with all antioxidant compounds, they actually become oxidizing compounds once their "good" work is done.

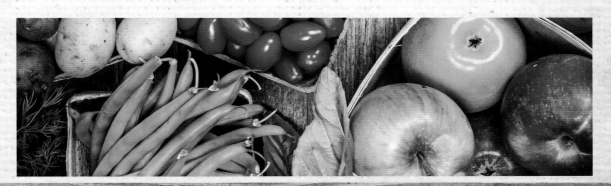

MEDICINAL MUSHROOMS

Evolution has given mankind any number of natural helpers. One of the natural substances used for the longest time is the mushroom. Quite a few varieties have been shown to have beneficial characteristics for human health and wellness. We know that more than 250 different species of mushrooms have been employed for therapeutic use throughout the ages. Traditional Chinese medicine has a particularly rich history of using a variety of species. About 100 such species are being actively studied by scientists today, with a handful of them (chaga, reishi, cordyceps, shiitake, maitake, lion's mane, and turkey tail, for example) rising above the rest for their health benefits.

The humble mushroom may not look impressive, but many species contain an impressive array of wellness-enhancing compounds.

A curious thing to note when considering the benefits of medicinal mushrooms is that humans are actually more closely related to fungi than to any other kingdom, including plants. Human beings share many of the same bacteria and viruses as mushrooms. When consuming medicinal mushrooms, then, the human body may recognize the natural antibiotics fungi have developed, and absorb them. Penicillin, streptomycin, and tetracycline all derive from fungal abstracts.

Many species of mushroom harvested in their natural habitats are known to hold properties beneficial to human health, including cancer-fighting and immunological properties. Some of the other studies focus on their use as antioxidants, liver protectors and cholesterol-lowering agents. Mushrooms may also contribute to human health as anti-diabetic, anti-inflammatory, anti-hypertensive, and antiviral agents.

The way mushrooms are cultivated can make a considerable difference in their ultimate medicinal effects. The innate ability of mushrooms to absorb nutrients has led some growers to enhance their mushrooms botanically by cultivating them within an organic environment containing immunity-supporting herbs. The method is thought by some to give such mushrooms even greater health- and wellness-enhancing qualities.

Fighting Cancer

Certain types of mushrooms produce immune cells that may be able to search out and destroy dangerous cancer cells. Back in an early era of Chinese folk medicine, *F. pinicola* was called out as an anticancer agent. Among more modern studies, its extracts have induced apoptosis in various human cancer cell lines and have inhibited tumor growth in some mice—promising test results that have scientists excited to learn more, an effort that is ongoing.

Enhancing Nutrition

Mushrooms in one's diet have been linked with improved overall nutrition. One study showed that eating dried, white button mushroom extract was as effective as taking supplemental vitamin D2 or D3 for raising vitamin D levels. Vitamin D intake has been known to help reduce the risk for cancer, heart disease, mood disorders, and bone loss. Numerous studies link the addition of mushrooms or mushroom extract to one's diet with better overall health and wellness.

Strengthening Immunity

Alkalizing the body and lowering inflammation have been associated with enhanced immunity and reduced disease risk. Not surprisingly, medicinal mushrooms may do both. The antibacterial compounds in mushrooms help them survive their environment, and isolating those compounds can be beneficial to human beings, too.

Helping the Heart

High cholesterol and hardening of the arteries are two risk factors for heart disease. Certain mushrooms produce compounds that have been linked to lowering cholesterol and keeping the arteries from hardening. They have also been linked to higher HDL— "good" cholesterol—levels, and their phytonutrients may help keep cells from sticking to blood vessel walls, which can improve circulation. These links between mushrooms and heart health are vast.

Boosting Energy and the Brain

Vitamin B compounds found in mushrooms support adrenal function, metabolism, and energy. They also may contribute to neurotransmitter and brain function, and possibly in the lowering of stress levels according to some studies. Clinical trials involving elderly patients have shown improvements in fatigue, cold intolerance, dizziness, and amnesia, among others. While further research on how mushrooms can lead to improvements in mood and help fight age-related neurodegenerative diseases is ongoing, the possible benefits could make a big impact on treatment and prevention programs.

Some physicians recommend adding 1-2 tablespoons of mushroom powder to food each day in order to boost health and wellness. Others recommend consuming mushrooms naturally, rather than as powders or supplements.

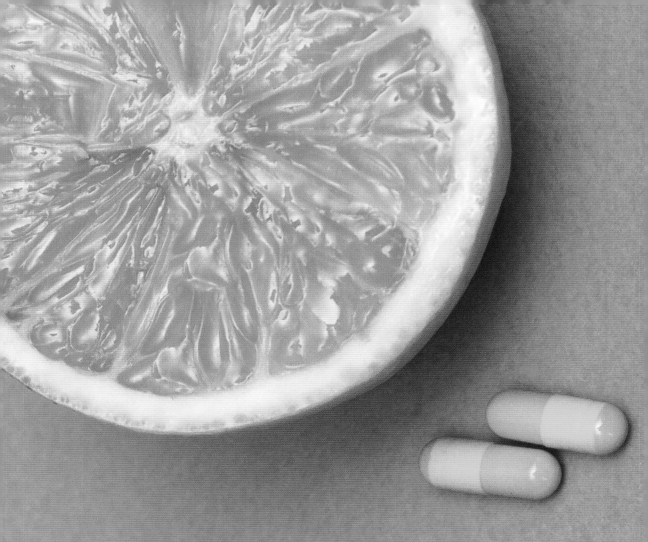

Natural
Antibiotics

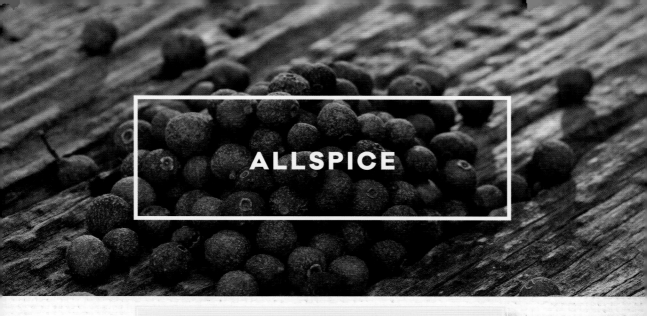

ALLSPICE

BOTANICAL NAME: *PIMENTA DIOICA*

Allspice derived its name from its unique aroma reminiscent of several different spices. The name was coined sometime in the early 17th century, thanks to its notes of cinnamon, clove, cardamom, nutmeg, and pepper. This versatile ingredient is a staple in Caribbean and Middle Eastern cuisine and can often be found in seasonal desserts in the U.S. But the plant's benefits go beyond food: the essential oil is prized for its many health uses.

Allspice is packed with antioxidants. The oil's antioxidant compounds include methyl eugenol and cineol, as well as vitamins A, B, and C. This makes it excellent for fighting oxidative stress in the body. In Jamaica, a folk remedy for the common cold involves drinking hot tea with plenty of allspice. The oil can be used to fight skin infections.

Spoil-inhibiting Standout

Allspice has traditionally been used to inhibit food spoilage. That tradition turns out to have solid scientific support. In one study, traditional food-preserving plants and spices were lab-tested to determine their efficacy. The results put allspice in the number three spot (out of 30). Here are the top 10:

1. Garlic
2. Onion
3. Allspice
4. Oregano
5. Thyme
6. Cinnamon
7. Tarragon
8. Cumin
9. Cloves
10. Lemongrass

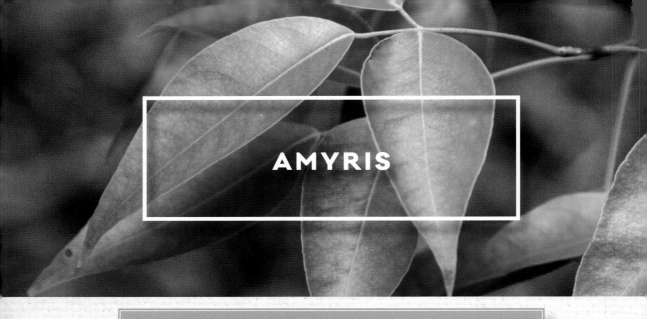

AMYRIS

BOTANICAL NAME: *AMYRIS BALSAMIFERA*

This evergreen tree grows in the wild mostly in Haiti and the Dominican Republic. The leaves and white flowers of the tree smell citrusy when they are crushed, and, in fact, the tree derived its name from the Greek word *amyron*, which means "intensely scented." Amyris is often also known as torchwood or candlewood, because the oil within the wood is highly combustible. The oil is extracted from the wood by steam distillation. It has a pleasant, sweetly woody and balsamic scent. Because of its attractive smell, amyris oil often shows up in soaps and perfumes, or is diffused to create a peaceful, relaxing atmosphere.

Another reason amyris appears in soaps is because of its antimicrobial properties. Amyris is very effective against acne, rashes, dry skin, and minor cuts and scrapes. It is also one of several essential oils that help repel ticks. It has been found to be effective against over 10 strains of multidrug-resistant bacteria like *Staphylococcus aureus* and *Salmonella paratyphi*.

TICK REPELLENT

Choose one:
2 parts either geranium or palmarosa oil

Choose one:
2 parts either amyris or Virginian cedarwood oil

Choose one:
1 part either vetiver or Alaskan cypress oil

Combine oils in a spray bottle in a base of distilled water. Try for a ratio of 5% oils to 95% water. Shake thoroughly before spraying on clothes.

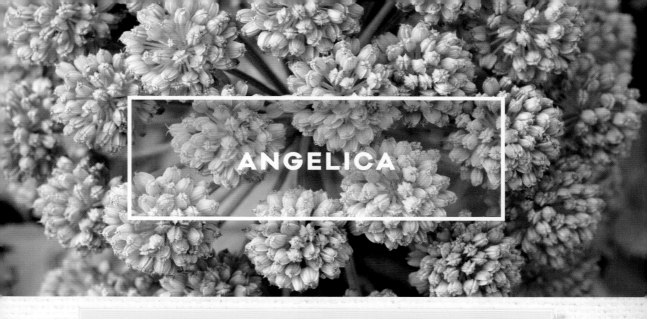

ANGELICA

BOTANICAL NAME: *ANGELICA ARCHANGELICA*

Commonly known as garden angelica, wild celery, or Norwegian angelica, this plant comes from the same family as carrots, parsnips, and fennel. The biennial plant—native to northern Europe and Greenland—is grown for its edible stems and sweet-smelling roots, which have been used medicinally since the 10th century. Its healing properties are so prized that the oil is also known as Holy Spirit Root, Archangel Root, and the Oil of Angels. Additionally, there are around 80 different aroma compounds found in angelica root, giving the essential oil its distinctive smell of musk and making it a favorite of perfumers and the food and beverage industry.

Angelica root's antispasmodic properties make it useful for relieving cramps, coughs, and muscle aches. It has been shown to be useful for treating gastritis, stomach ulcers, gas, and indigestion. Angelica essential oil has a lovely fragrance on its own, and it also blends well with other essential oils; this makes it excellent for use in calming aromatherapy. The root is antibacterial and can be applied as a natural food preservative.

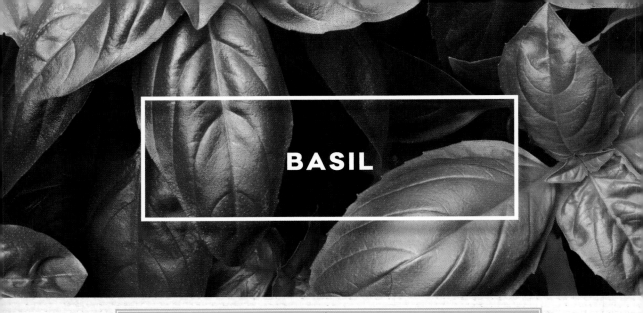

BASIL

BOTANICAL NAME: *OCIMUM BASILICUM*

Named after the Greek *basileus*, meaning "king," basil—the "king of herbs"—has been cultivated in India for at least 5,000 years. It has been used for culinary purposes in Asian and Mediterranean cultures for centuries, and today many of us know it mostly as an essential pizza and pesto ingredient. But the tasty herb was often used in ancient Chinese and Ayurvedic medicinal practices to treat coughs, fevers, indigestion, constipation, and skin rashes. The herb is also used in religious practices in the Eastern Orthodox Church and Hinduism. The spicy, herby scented oil can be diluted in olive or coconut oil and applied topically, or used in a diffuser.

Basil is broadly antibacterial, antiviral, analgesic, and an insect repellent. Research has shown that basil oil is effective at fighting bacteria and fungi, making it an excellent choice for a natural kitchen and bathroom cleaner. The oil also helps to kill odor-causing bacteria and mold on furniture, kitchen appliances, or in your car. You can use the oil when fighting colds or the flu by diffusing it in your home, or adding a few drops to a bath. Try adding a few drops of basil oil to coconut oil and rubbing into sore, painful muscles. The oil can also be used to make bug repellent, mouthwash, or toothpaste.

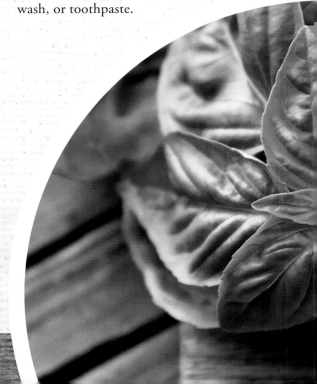

Basil and Vinegar Surface Cleaner

This simple and organic recipe provides a great way to clean countertops of germs. A few minutes after use, the vinegar smell will fade, leaving behind the fresh scent of basil.

In a large glass jar add 8 ounces white vinegar, 4 ounces water, and 1 cup loose fresh basil. Close jar tightly and refrigerate for several weeks. When ready, strain the vinegar infusion into a spray bottle. Spray and wipe as needed.

Have you ever wondered why basil shows up in a multitude of cleaning products? It's not included just for its pleasant odor. Basil kills quite a few common kitchen pathogens. In one study, basil was tested against *S. aureus, E. coli, B. subtilis, Pasteurella multocida, A. niger, Mucor mucedo, F. solani, Botryodiplodia theobromae,* and *R. solani.* The results were spectacular. Basil showed strong antimicrobial activity against all tested microorganisms. Basil extract also performed well against the bacterial species *B. cereus, Micrococcus flavus, S. aureus* and *E. faecalis, P. aeruginosa, S. typhimurium,* and *L. monocytogenes* and the fungi *A. fumigatus, A. niger, A. versicolor, A. ochraceus, Penicillium funiculosum, Penicillium ochrochloron,* and *Trichoderma viride.* The essential oil tends to be even more efficacious than an extract.

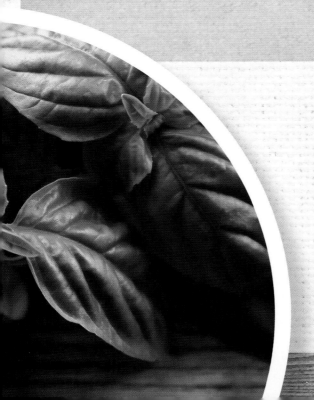

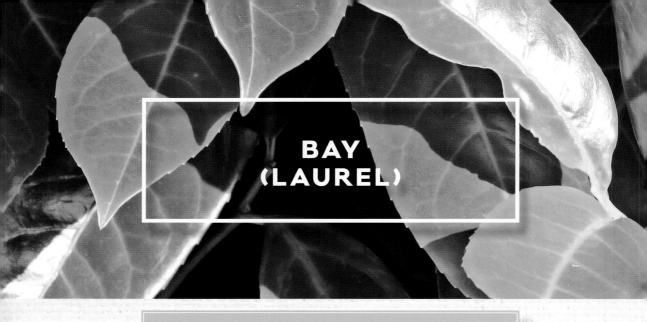

BAY (LAUREL)

BOTANICAL NAME: *LAURUS NOBILIS*

The leaves of the bay laurel plant are probably best known via the kitchen spice rack. Dried bay leaves are used as flavoring agents in soups and stocks in many cuisines. But traditionally, the plant had medicinal uses as well. It was used to alleviate stomach ailments, and the essential oil has been used to create the famous "Aleppo soap" since antiquity. Today, the ornamental plant is still popular in the Mediterranean region, and the essential oil distilled from its aromatic leaves is prized for its many health benefits and spicy scent.

The essential oil is antiseptic, antibacterial, analgesic, and helps to relieve symptoms of colds and flu (especially achy muscles). It has even been used as an insecticide. Lab tests have shown bay to be an effective antifungal.

Remedy for Acne

Bay leaf is a traditional remedy for acne. Its antiseptic and antibacterial properties, along with its high antioxidant content makes it effective at killing acne-causing germs. Bay also has skin-soothing and rejuvenating properties. One of the simplest ways to use bay against acne is to prepare a tea (simmer a handful of leaves in water for 20 minutes), let the tea cool, and rinse your face with the liquid. Using bay leaf in steam treatments, tinctures, and tonics is also common in home remedies.

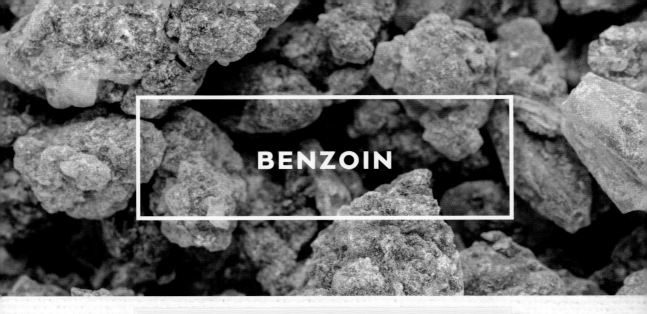

BENZOIN

BOTANICAL NAME: *STYRAX BENZOIN*

The trunk of the benzoin tree exudes a vanilla-scented gum resin when cut. Used since antiquity in medicine, it was imported by the Arabs to use as a less expensive substitute for frankincense. They made pomades that smelled like vanilla and were rubbed on the skin for fragrance and healing. Traders brought benzoin to Greece, Rome, and Egypt, where it became prized as a fixative in perfumes—still one of its uses today. Europeans highly regarded benzoin for its medicinal properties as well as its scent. The essential oil is typically sold as an absolute, but it is so thick it may be difficult for you to get it out of the bottle. If so, dilute it with a little alcohol or dissolve it in warm carrier oil so it is easier to pour.

Benzoin is an antibacterial, antifungal, antioxidant, and anti-inflammatory. It helps to seal wounds from infection. One of its most popular uses is in a cream to protect chapped skin and improve skin elasticity. Since it is a strong preservative, adding it to vegetable oil-based preparations delays their oxidation and spoilage. Benzoin essential oil can be added to chest rub balms and massage oils for lung and sinus ailments.

Benzoin Tincture

Benzoin tincture is available in over-the-counter form. It may be used topically for skin problems and canker sores. It is also mixed with hot water to provide a steam inhalant. The U.S. military has used it to treat blisters. After a blister is drained, the tincture is injected into the void, sanitizing the wound and gluing the skin together. Benzoin is a major component of Friar's Balsam, a traditional remedy used both topically (for cuts, abrasions, chapped skin, and bedsores) and as an inhalant (as a stimulating expectorant for coughs, flu, laryngitis, bronchitis, and asthma).

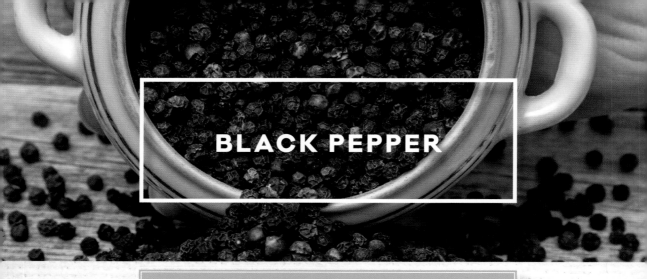

BLACK PEPPER

BOTANICAL NAME: *PIPER NIGRUM*

Traded more than any other spice in the world, black pepper has been prized since antiquity not only for its flavor-enhancing spiciness, but also for its medicinal usefulness. The spice has been found in ancient Egyptian tombs, was frequently used in ancient Roman cook ery, and was so coveted by Europeans that it was briefly used as a form of currency. In fact, Alaric the Visigoth, famous for sacking the city of Rome in the year 410, demanded 3,000 pounds of pepper as a ransom for the city! The spice is obtained by cooking and drying the unripe fruit of the flowering vine. Once dried, oil can be extracted from the fruit by crushing it.

The warming properties of black pepper oil make it ideal for soothing sore muscles and aiding in relief from arthritis and rheumatism. A couple diluted drops rubbed into the affected area can help improve pain and ease mobility. Taken internally (again, diluted), black pepper oil protects the body from free radicals and helps to repair cell damage, and has even been shown to lower cholesterol.

Quick Relief for the Common Cold

Pepper tea anyone? Believe it or not, pepper has been used to make tea for centuries. In this form, it is credited with the ability to relieve headaches, alleviate sore throats, and ease gastrointestinal distress. It was also believed to increase saliva flow and stimulate the appetite. It is undoubtedly a sinus-clearing remedy for respiratory issues. Whip this up quickly when you're feeling congested or sneezy:

- 2 cups water
- 1 teaspoon fresh grated black pepper
- Juice of ½ lemon
- 1 teaspoon honey (optional)

Add all ingredients to saucepan, bring to a boil, and pour in cup. Drink this concoction when it has become lukewarm.

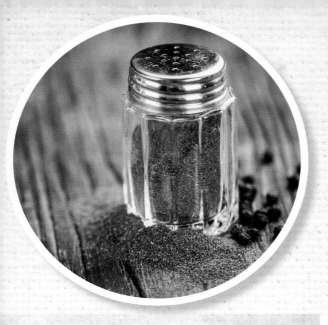

Black pepper begins as a cluster of green fruit on a flowering vine. *Piper nigrum* is native to the southwestern region of India. The still-green fruits—known as *drupes*—are briefly cooked in hot water before drying in the sun for several days. This process oxidizes the outer layer (the pericarp), turning it black. When the pericarp is removed during processing, the result is white pepper. Both white and black pepper contain similar amounts of piperine, one of the medicinal compounds in the spice.

Black pepper is an excellent digestive aid. Not only does it stimulate digestive enzymes and tone the digestive tract, it also optimizes the body's ability to absorb nutrients. One study showed that growths of *E. coli* and *S. aureus* bacteria were inhibited by the introduction of black pepper. But plenty of anecdotal evidence suggests that black pepper's antibacterial properties are broad spectrum—by consuming black pepper, you are giving your immune system a general antibacterial, anti-inflammatory, antioxidant boost.

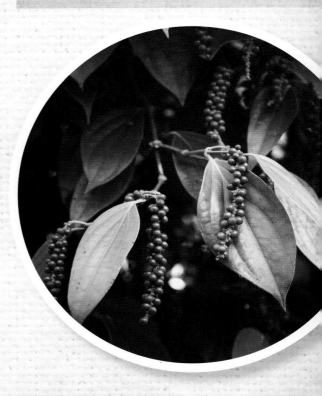

Staphylococcus aureus is a major problem in hospitals due to its resistance to common antibiotics. Recent studies prove that extracts of black pepper are very effective at reducing colonies of this pathogen.

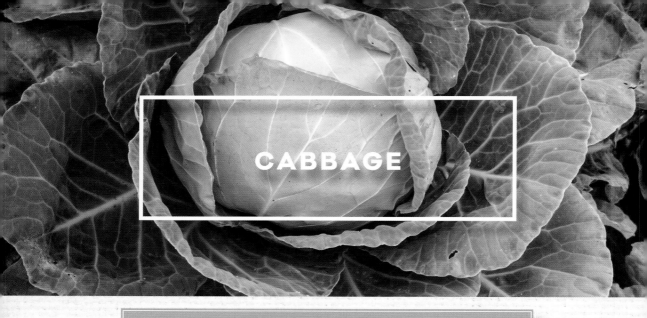

CABBAGE

BOTANICAL NAME: *BRASSICA OLERACEA*

Cabbage may lack the glamor of some superfoods, but this humble vegetable actually boasts incredible health benefits and antibiotic properties. It is rich in sulfur and vitamin C, making it perfect as a defense against common ailments. Cabbage is a member of the *Brassicaceae* family, which includes Brussels sprouts, cauliflower, kohlrabi, and broccoli.

Cabbage is one of the oldest cultivated vegetables and may have been domesticated over 2,500 years ago. In its original form, the plant did not form a round head of leaves. The first cabbages looked similar to kale. Its wild ancestor was native to parts of the eastern Mediterranean and the Middle East. Its health benefits were touted by a number of Roman writers.

While cabbage is already healthy in its raw form, fermented cabbage (for example, sauerkraut and kimchi) is truly a probiotic powerhouse. The lactic acid bacteria used to make sauerkraut helps to improve intestinal tract health and immunity.

Cabbage juice has been used to prevent and heal ulcers for more than 40 years. Current research at the Stanford University School of Medicine revealed that when ulcer patients drank 1 quart of raw cabbage juice each day, ulcers in the stomach and small intestine healed in about five days. People who ate cabbage instead of drinking the juice also had faster healing times than those who did not eat cabbage. Cabbage accomplishes this by killing bacteria, including the ulcer-causing *H. pylori*. Secondly, it contains a phytochemical called gefarnate that coaxes stomach cells into making extra mucus, which protects the stomach wall from digestive acid.

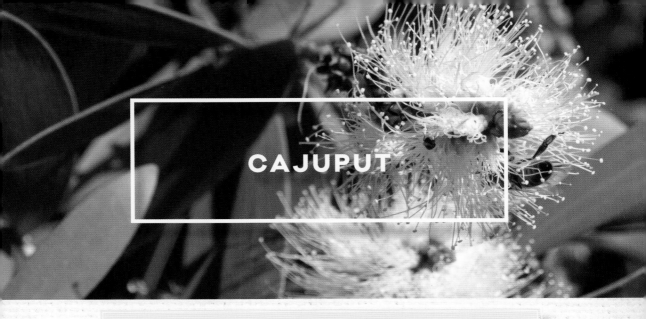

CAJUPUT

BOTANICAL NAME: *MELALEUCA CAJUPUTI*

Found mainly in Australia, Southeast Asia, and New Guinea, the cajuput tree has been used as a source of healing ingredients for centuries. Aboriginal Australians discovered that the leaves of the tree could be employed to treat aches and pains. They would also crush the leaves and inhale the vapors to ease respiratory ailments. And in Asia, the leaves have been used to make comforting herbal teas and therapeutic liniments.

Today, Cajuput essential oil is distilled from the leaves and twigs of the tree, and is often compared to tea tree oil. The oil has a pungent, camphor-like smell, with an herby undertone reminiscent of rosemary. It has a pleasant warming property that is excellent for soothing sore muscles; but that's just one of its many benefits. Topically, cajuput is an antibacterial, antifungal, and antiviral. It is also an excellent pest repellent.

Cajuput is a great addition to a first aid kit due to its antiseptic properties. It can be applied to cuts and wounds to ward off bacterial, fungal, and viral infections, and can also be used to clear up acne or to treat skin conditions like psoriasis. Used in an inhaler, cajuput helps relieve congestion due to colds and flu. The oil's warming effects make it perfect for soothing achy, sore muscles, and it helps to improve circulation. Cajuput oil can be diluted in a carrier oil and rubbed on the skin to repel insects, or it can be sprayed around your home to keep out unwanted critters.

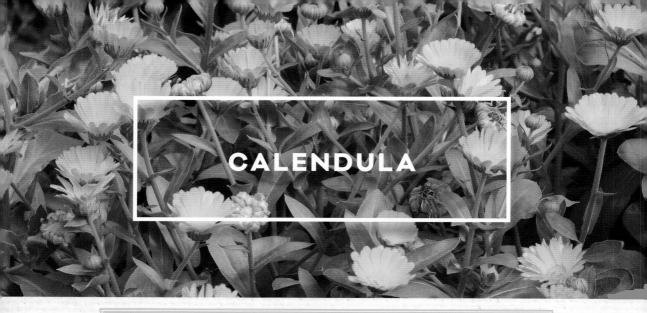

CALENDULA

BOTANICAL NAME: *CALENDULA OFFICINALIS*

Calendula—often referred to as the pot marigold—is an edible flower that has been used for centuries in European, Middle Eastern, and Mediterranean cooking. The bright yellow petals were sometimes used to add color to butter and cheese, or as a fabric dye. But calendula's usefulness goes far beyond its taste and color: the flower is mentioned in some of history's earliest medical texts, where it was recommended for aiding digestion, preventing infections, and detoxifying the liver. The flower was even used on the battlefield during the Civil War and World War I, as a remedy to prevent infection of open wounds. The sticky, syrupy oil distilled from the flowers is often extracted by steeping the petals in a hot carrier oil.

Calendula is a potent remedy for many inflammatory ailments, including dermatitis, ear infections, sore throats, ulcers, and diaper rash. Its muscle-relaxing properties can be used for abdominal cramps or constipation, and provide relief from PMS symptoms. It is also a popular additive in toothpastes, mouthwashes, and topical antiseptic ointments, due to its powerful antimicrobial properties. Note, however, that some people are allergic to calendula and other related plants, including ragweed, chamomile, and echinacea. Due to its muscle-relaxing properties, there is a possibility that it could interact negatively with some medications, including sedatives and diabetes or blood pressure medication. Pregnant women should also avoid calendula.

As a medicinal herb, calendula has been used in Europe since at least the 12th century. But even before that, it was revered by a number of civilizations. The name comes from the Latin *calends* (meaning the first day of the month), possibly because the Romans thought it would always bloom at this time. The ancient Greeks used it as a culinary garnish. The ancient Egyptians used the sap to heal wounds and help the skin regenerate. In fact, stylized calendula flowers appear in hieroglyphics that are thousands of years old.

Homegrown Medicine

Calendula is easy to grow. The seeds are sown in ground that gets plenty of sun in mid-spring. Two weeks after germination, the plants are thinned to about 12 inches apart. Calendula is harvested when the flowers are at full bloom. The entire flower heads can be harvested and dried. Once fully dried, they are best stored in airtight glass jars or sealed plastic bags.

The dried flowers can be used in endless ways: teas, infusions, tinctures, salves, or prepared in meals. A simple way to take advantage of calendula's antibiotic properties in topical applications is to add flowers to a canning jar about halfway and fill to the top with a carrier oil. Cap the jar and store in a dark place 4-6 weeks, shaking occasionally. Applied to the skin, this infusion has soothing, antibiotic, anti-inflammatory, and healing properties.

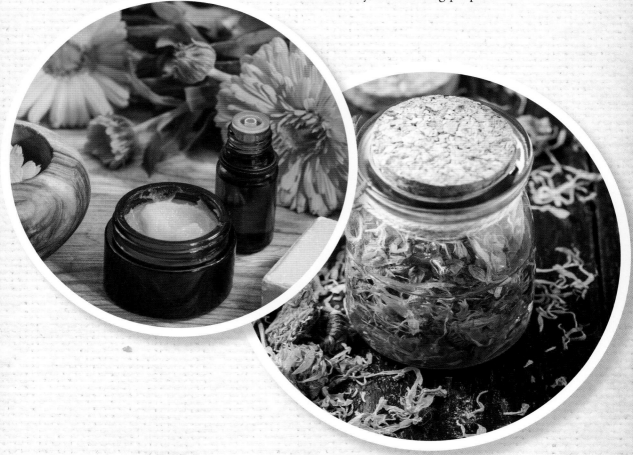

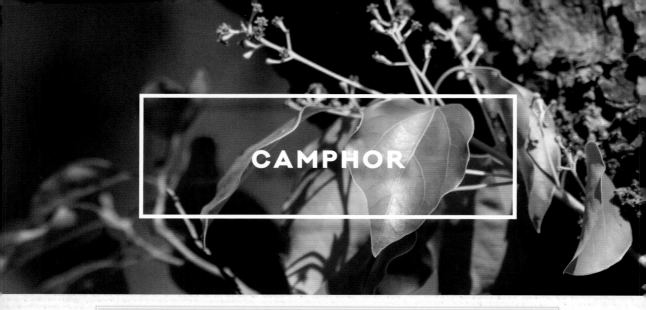

CAMPHOR

BOTANICAL NAME: *CINNAMOMUM CAMPHORA*

The camphor laurel is a large evergreen tree native to China, Japan, and other Asian countries. In fact, the third largest tree ever documented in Japan is an 82-foot-tall camphor laurel, which is said to have first sprouted in prehistoric times. The wood and leaves of these trees are steam distilled to extract the essential oil, which has been used for centuries in everything from embalming fluid to medicines to insect repellent. Although researchers can't trace the first time the oil was ever used, they suspect that its strong scent and decongestant properties are what cemented camphor's place as a medicinal mainstay.

Camphor is popularly used as a decongestant because of its strong, sinus-clearing scent. It is also an excellent disinfectant, and can be added to ointments and lotions to aid skin conditions and kill bacteria. It provides a cooling sensation to the skin, making it ideal for mixing with bath water to escape oppressive summer heat. It works well to repel and kill unwanted insects.

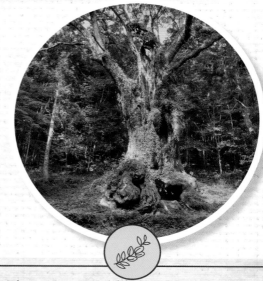

This 3,000-year-old sacred camphor tree grows in Takeo Shrine, on Japan's southern island Kyushu. It is one of the largest in the country. The tree is venerated in Japan. Historically the wood has been prized for making pest-repelling furniture.

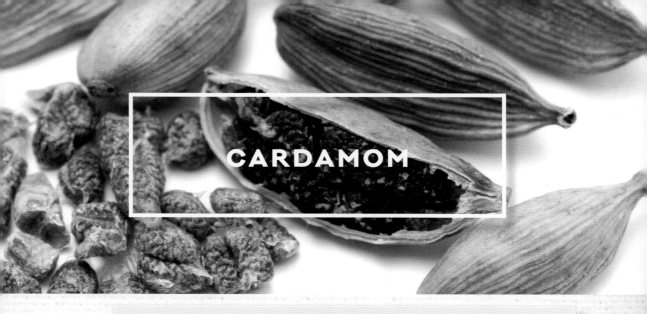

CARDAMOM

BOTANICAL NAME: *ELETTARIA CARDAMOMUM*

If you've ever sipped a cup of spicy chai tea or enjoyed Arabic coffee, your beverage was probably flavored with a healthy dose of cardamom. The third most expensive spice in the world—only vanilla and saffron surpass it—cardamom is native to India. The fragrant spice has soothing properties that make it great for aiding digestion and calming stomach upset. Try inhaling the scent on car or boat trips to ward off motion sickness. Sniffing the essential oil can help relieve anxiety and promote feelings of calm.

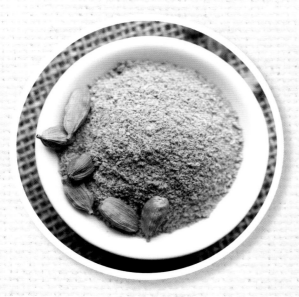

Better oral and digestive health may be as simple as chewing on a cardamom pod. In India, cardamom has a long history as a traditional healing component for intestinal maladies. It has been used to fight bacterial infections in the colon and stomach, to combat *H. pylori*, and for curing urinary tract infections. Studies seem to bear out its antimicrobial reputation. The essential oil is effective at inhibiting the growth and spread of bacterial pathogens. And one recent study showed that a simple cardamom extract was effective against oral bacteria like *Streptococcus mutans* and *Candida albicans*.

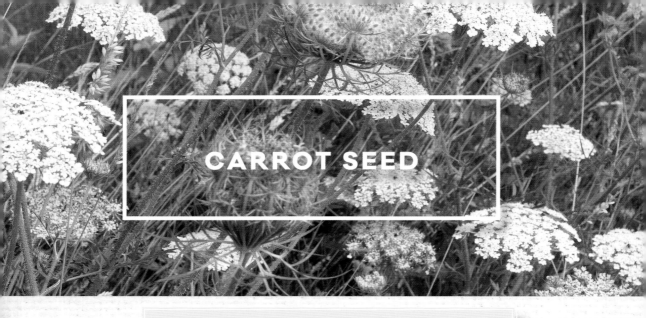

CARROT SEED

BOTANICAL NAME: *DAUCUS CAROTA*

Carrot seed, in this context, refers to the wild, rather than the domestic, carrot. This flowering plant is also known as Queen Anne's Lace. The essential oil is readily available and is considered to be one of the hidden stars of the medicinal essential oils. Carrot seed oil can be applied topically, either on its own or mixed with lotion or face cream, to rejuvenate skin or help ward off infections. When diluted and ingested, it seems to help fight infections of the mouth and digestive system. It can help treat colds, the flu, and bronchitis. Its soothing aroma helps relieve stress and anxiety when used in aromatherapy. The oil even helps kill intestinal parasites, but is safely consumed by humans. Carrot seed should not be ingested by pregnant women however, as it is an abortifacient.

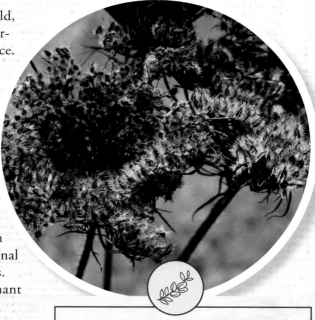

Carrot seed was prized in ancient times for its ability to aid digestion and soothe stomach ailments.

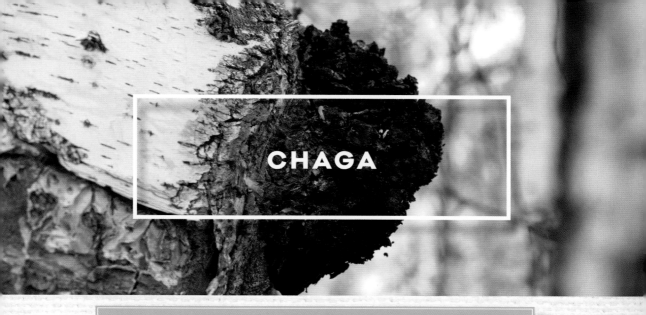

CHAGA

The undisputed "king of the medicinal mushrooms," chaga has been used for thousands of years by native tribes and indigenous people across Europe, Asia, and North America as an across-the-board health booster. Historical records from 17th-century Russia indicate it was used to battle gastrointestinal issues, various forms of cancer, and many, many ailments in between. In Finland, chaga tea has been brewed for centuries.

Chaga mushrooms prefer growing on birch trees in the cooler climates of the northern United States, Canada, and northern Europe and Asia. Chaga does not look much like a "traditional" mushroom. It's rather a hardened, black, crusty growth on the birch that can resemble charcoal. Inside the crust is a soft, orange-colored core.

Chaga's unique structure makes it more conducive for ingesting as a prepared powder, a brewed drink, or a supplement than as a mushroom to be eaten. It is extremely tough and chitinous—eating it would be like trying to eat tree bark. When it is prepared at home, a long brewing time at low temperature is typically required.

Its use in traditional cultures to fight a wide range of ailments has been borne out by research. There is evidence that chaga aids in numerous health-boosting efforts and can help ward off a number of health issues.

What follows is just a brief look at some of its many therapeutic uses.

Cancer Prevention and Treatment

Perhaps the most touted use of chaga is in the prevention and treatment of various forms of cancer. The mushroom's high levels of antioxidants, including triterpene, are thought to be the primary reason for its effects in this area. Antioxidants are known to protect cells from damage by free radicals, and triterpene in particular has been successful in test-tube studies in killing cancer cells while not harming healthy cells. Other test-tube studies have shown that chaga extract may be able to prevent the growth of cancer in liver cells, with similar results also seen against cancer cells of the breast, lungs, colon, and prostate. In a 2010 study, chaga slowed the growth of lung, breast, and cervical cancer cells in a petri dish and was able to slow the growth of tumors in mice. Although the antioxidants in chaga are undeniable and much of the research is promising, it is important to keep in mind that these studies have largely been done in laboratory environments.

Inflammation and the Immune System

When the body's immune system is under attack, inflammation is often the result. The body becomes temporarily inflamed in an effort to ward off illness and disease. However, long-term inflammation can become a chronic health problem of its own, including links to such conditions as inflammatory bowel disease (IBD) or rheumatoid arthritis (RA). Chaga mushrooms have displayed some therapeutic success here. According to a 2007 study published in *Biofactors*, using chaga extract to treat cells from 20 healthy volunteers along with 20 volunteers diagnosed with IBD helped reduce oxidative stress—a process thought to contribute to IBD development.

Chaga has been shown to promote the formation of helpful cytokines, beneficial proteins that help regulate the immune system. By doing so, chaga may stimulate the white blood cells that play a critical role in battling bacteria and viruses ranging from common colds to serious diseases.

Heart Disease

The antioxidants in chaga mushrooms may reduce LDL (bad) cholesterol that can contribute to heart disease. In an eight-week study of rats with high LDL cholesterol, chaga extract did just that. Several other studies have produced similar results while also linking the chaga boost to higher HDL (good) cholesterol numbers. There is considerable thought that these same antioxidants, along with perhaps the betulinic acid found in chaga, might have helpful impacts on high blood pressure—another condition associated with heart disease.

Aging

Of course, no mushroom (or medicine, for that matter) can turn back the clock on actual aging. For some of the common signs of aging like wrinkles, sagging skin and gray hair, though, some swear by the chaga mushroom as a fungal fountain of youth. Some aging signs are caused by oxidative stress or free radicals in the body, sometimes attributed to sun exposure, pollution, or other stressors that accelerate the skin's aging process. Studies have shown chaga, in some circumstances, to be effective against oxidative stress and free radicals.

Others

There may be a case to add diabetes to the list at some point. In a 2006 study over an eight-week period, chaga was able to lower the blood sugar of rats that were modified to be obese and have diabetes. There have been no human studies to compare to those findings, so much research lies ahead. There is also some early evidence that chaga can help combat some side effects of other treatments, including chemotherapy and radiation. Though further testing is needed, the "king of the medicinal mushrooms" has been widely lauded around the world for its health- and wellness-boosting prowess and its potential ability to fight off many common and more serious health concerns. Extracts and teas from chaga mushrooms have become especially popular. It should be noted, however, that some have experienced side effects from chaga. Its impact on blood sugar might be dangerous for those on insulin or with diabetes. Those with autoimmune diseases should consult a doctor before adding chaga due to the mushroom's potential to stimulate the immune system. The same is true for those pregnant or breastfeeding.

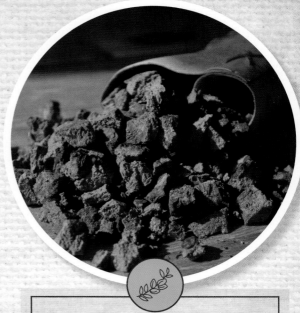

After harvest, chaga may be cut into smaller chunks and directly decocted. However, the smaller the pieces, the easier it is to extract the bioactive ingredients. For this reason, the chunks are often ground into a powder.

Looks can be deceiving. The ugly black "crust" around chaga contains a high concentration of melanin. It may also contain up to 30 percent betulin. Herbal practitioners note that it is important to include this layer when making decoctions, as it seems to confer immunity-enhancing benefits, especially against the flu virus.

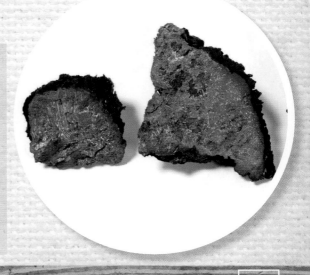

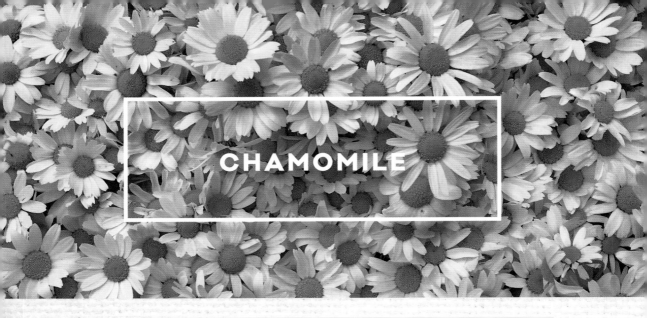

CHAMOMILE

BOTANICAL NAME: *MATRICARIA CHAMOMILLA (GERMAN), CHAMAEMELUM NOBILE (ROMAN)*

Varieties of chamomile have been used medicinally for thousands of years. Ancient Egyptians used it to treat nervous afflictions and sleeping problems. Ancient Romans used it to treat skin and respiratory conditions. It takes its name from the Greek word *chamaimelon*, meaning "ground apple." Greek physicians treated intestinal disorders with chamomile. During the Middle Ages it was used to treat a variety of ailments and was also used as a strewing herb—bundles of the plant were simply thrown on the floor where they would be walked over, releasing their scent, repelling vermin, and helping to clear the air. One Anglo-Saxon manuscript tells us that chamomile was one of the "Nine Sacred Herbs." Modern herbalists continue to recommend chamomile for many of its traditional uses. Medieval monks planted raised garden beds of chamomile, and those who were sad or depressed lay on them as therapy.

Chamomile flowers resemble daisies, but one sniff will have you thinking of apples instead. Inhaling chamomile tea's aroma relaxes both the mind and the body. Research studies show that chamomile relaxes emotions, muscles, and even brain waves. It eases the emotional ups and downs of PMS, menopause, and hyperactivity in children. It also helps control the pain of bruises, stiff joints, headaches, sore muscles, menstrual and digestive system cramping, as well as the pain and swelling of sprains and some allergic reactions. Chamomile is mild enough to ease a baby's colic and calm it for sleep. It is especially soothing in a massage oil, as a compress, or in a bath. Make a chamomile room spray by diluting 12 drops of the essential oil per ounce of distilled water. Chamomile is suitable for most complexion types or skin problems, from burns and eczema to varicose veins. It is especially useful for sensitive, puffy, or inflamed conditions. Drinking chamomile tea after meals settles the stomach.

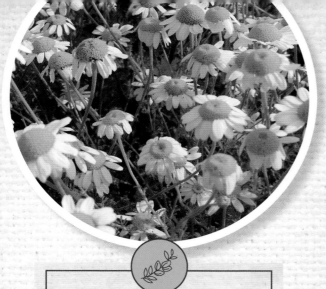

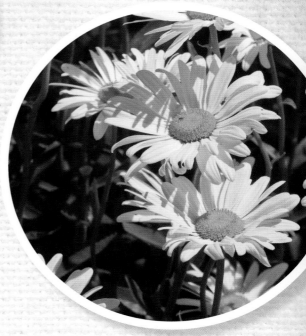

Similar in appearance, but with somewhat different healing properties, German chamomile (above) and Roman chamomile (right) can both be used to calm and relax the nervous system.

The striking blue to blue-green color of German chamomile's essential oil comes from chamazulene. This powerful compound can also be found in a few other essential oils, like blue tansy, wormwood, and yarrow. Chamazulene's healing properties are truly amazing. Thanks to its ability to fight inflammation and infection and promote tissue regeneration, this compound is applicable to just about any common skin condition. Chamazulene is helpful in dealing with eczema, psoriasis, dermatitis, poison ivy, cuts, infections, boils, blisters, warts, insect bites, sunburn, and even deeper tissue ailments, from surface bruises to rheumatic pain.

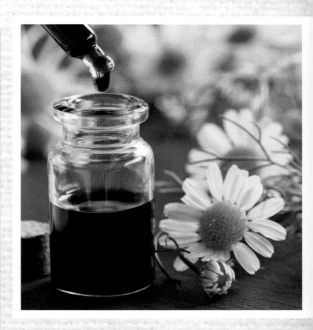

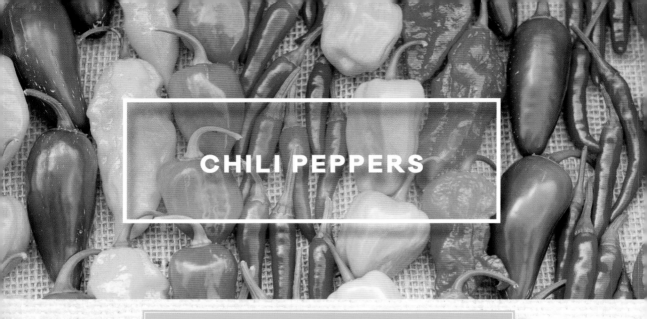

CHILI PEPPERS

BOTANICAL NAME: *CAPSICUM*

Human use of chili peppers goes back to prehistoric times. Archaeological and historical evidence points to South American chili usage going back at least 5,000 years. Domestication probably began even earlier—maybe 6,500 years ago—in central-east Mexico. Chili peppers were restricted to the Americas for most of their existence, but the arrival of European explorers signaled their global spread. Europeans brought chilis back to Europe, where they made inroads in southern European cooking. The Portuguese took chilis with them to multiple points in Africa and India. Chilis spread quickly to Indonesia, China, and Japan. In fact, few other foods have been adopted so quickly by so many people.

It is estimated that 50,000 chili pepper cultivars exist. This should give some indication of how valued they are across the globe.

Obviously, they add spice and flavor to other foods, but chilis are packed with benefits that go far beyond the culinary. It was probably noticed early on that chilis helped reduce food spoilage—chilis naturally evolved the ability to repel microbes—and this was extremely valuable in the days before refrigeration. And wherever food spoilage lurks, the risk of food poisoning increases. One study showed that a crude extract of chili stopped cholera bacteria from producing toxins. Other studies indicate that chili extracts will inhibit or kill a number of bacteria (*H. pylori* and *P. aeruginosa*, for example) depending on the dosage. Obtaining consistent results is difficult, though. There are hundreds of varieties of chili peppers to utilize and their respective bioactive compounds are not well understood.

Cayenne

Although it can set your mouth on fire, cayenne, ironically, is good for your digestive system and is now known to help heal ulcers. It reduces substance P, a chemical that carries pain messages from the skin's nerve endings, so it reduces pain when applied topically. A cayenne cream is now in use to treat psoriasis, postsurgical pain, shingles, and nerve damage from diabetes.

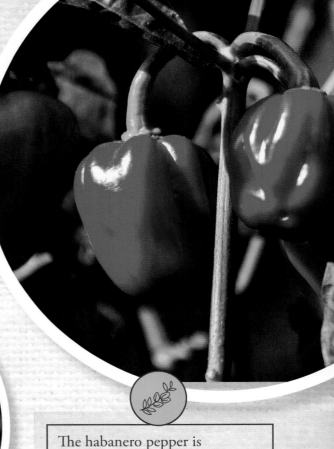

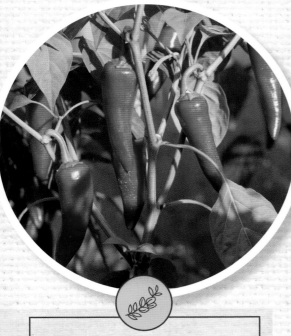

Cayenne's red podlike fruits are extremely hot. Cayenne grows naturally in the tropics, but gardeners in most parts of the United States can grow it with success.

The habanero pepper is particularly hot, having an abundance of capsaicin. However, habaneros do not seem to be as effective against bacteria as some other pepper varieties. In fact, milder jalapenos seem to be better at stopping or killing bacteria. Some compounds responsible for the antimicrobial properties of chili peppers remain a mystery.

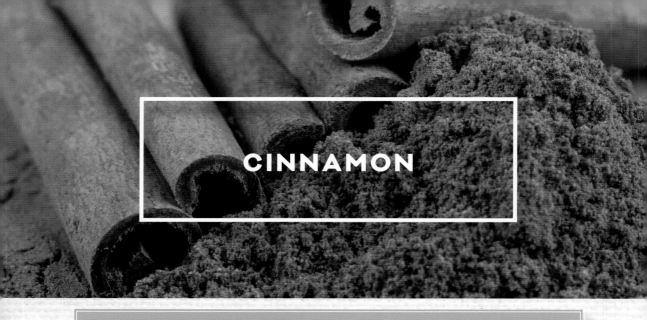

CINNAMON

BOTANICAL NAME: *CINNAMOMUM ZEYLANICUM*

The zeylanicum "true" cinnamon starts off as the dry inner bark of a large, 20-to-30-foot tree. Cinnamon flavors mouthwashes, foods, and drinks. Cinnamon's scent stirs the appetite, invigorates and "warms" the senses, and may even produce a feeling of joy. Although it is used primarily as a food spice, cinnamon is a powerful antibacterial as well. Both the extract and essential oil show high activity against a wide variety of bacteria. Cinnamon is also a potent antiviral: a simple mixture of honey and cinnamon mixed into water provides excellent support against respiratory ailments like colds and coughs. In a study conducted by a group of surgeons, cinnamon oil proved an effective antiseptic against hospital-acquired infections like MRSA.

Who knew tree bark could be an all-purpose panacea? Researchers have found that it also reduces drowsiness, irritability, and the pain and number of headaches. The essential oil and its fragrance help relax tight muscles, ease painful joints, and relieve menstrual cramps. Historically, the Chinese have used it to treat inflammatory conditions, gastrointestinal disorders, and urinary infections.

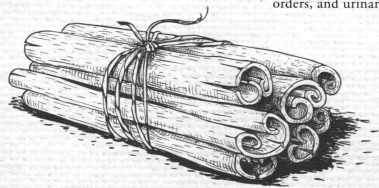

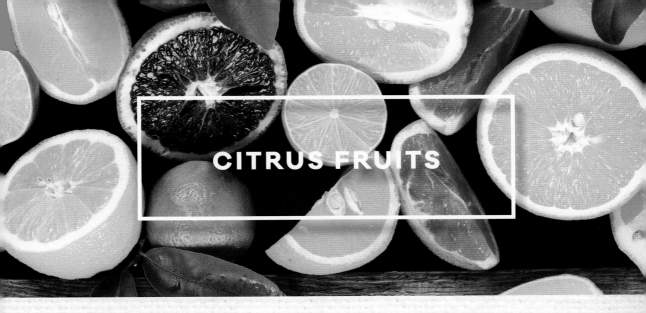

CITRUS FRUITS

The fruits of the citrus family are diverse, and so are their protective benefits. They are broadly antimicrobial in their natural state and as essential oils. The flavonoids alone are antibacterial, antifungal, and antiviral. One simple molecule present in many citrus fruits, limonene, is strongly antiviral. Simply put, if you're eating citrus, you're eating a natural antibiotic. If you're cleaning with citrus, you're cleaning with a natural antibiotic.

Herbal healing methods often employ citrus peels, particularly as a component of tea blends. The simple technique of steeping unlocks powerful antimicrobial compounds like limonene, myrcene, pinene, thujene, and citral. When doing this, make sure you're using organic peels, to avoid hard-to-remove pesticide residue.

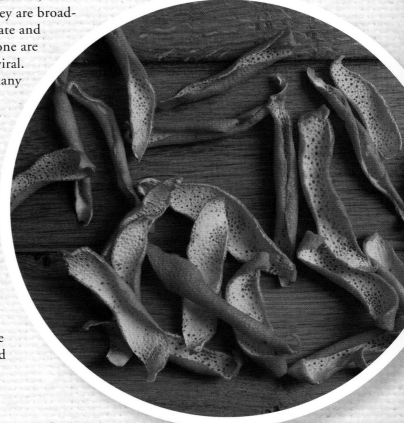

Bergamot

BOTANICAL NAME:
CITRUS BERGAMIA

The same small citrus fruit used to flavor Earl Grey tea is also a potent antimicrobial. Bergamot fights several viruses, including those that cause flu, herpes, shingles, and chicken pox. Due to its versatile antibiotic properties, it also treats bacterial infections of the urinary system, mouth, and throat. It is helpful for a variety of skin conditions, including eczema. As a natural deodorant, it not only provides a pleasant scent, but it kills bacteria that are responsible for odor.

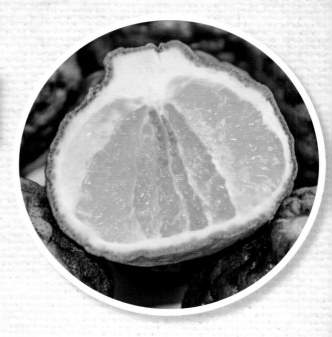

Lemon

BOTANICAL NAME:
CITRUS LIMONUM

The common lemon is an antimicrobial miracle worker. Studies show that the oil increases the activity of the immune system by stimulating the production of the white corpuscles that fight infection. Additionally, lemon essential oil counters a wide range of viral and bacterial infections. Massage it on the skin in a carrier oil base to relieve congested lymph glands. Add lemon juice to your daily diet to fight off colds and the flu.

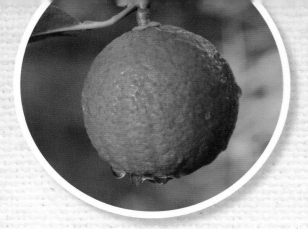

Orange

BOTANICAL NAME: CITRUS SINENSIS

Although not as antibiotic as lemon, don't overlook the common orange. It has value in fighting the flu, colds, and breaking up congested lymph, especially when added to massage oil. As a kitchen cleaner, orange oil is very effective, and it smells fantastic! It will inhibit the spread of *E. coli* and *salmonella*. It's effective against many fungal strains. Many studies have demonstrated its effectiveness, but to list just one: a 1996 study tested orange oil against 22 strains of bacteria. It inhibited all of them.

Lime

BOTANICAL NAME: CITRUS AURANTIFOLIA

Lime oil has been shown to protect against infections in minor cuts and scrapes, as well as ward off colds and flu. It works well to heal skin conditions such as psoriasis, rashes, and acne. As with lemon juice, simply adding the juice to your diet may be enough to ward off common seasonal ailments.

Mandarin

BOTANICAL NAME: CITRUS RETICULATA

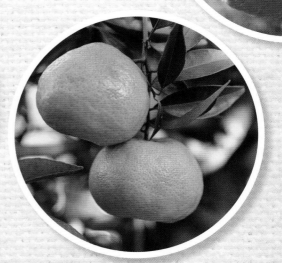

Mandarin oil protects wounds from infection, and is also especially good at protecting food from bacterial growth. It helps to prevent acne and diminishes the appearance of stretch marks and scars. Thanks to its antimicrobial properties and great scent, the oil is perfect to use as a natural household cleaner and air freshener.

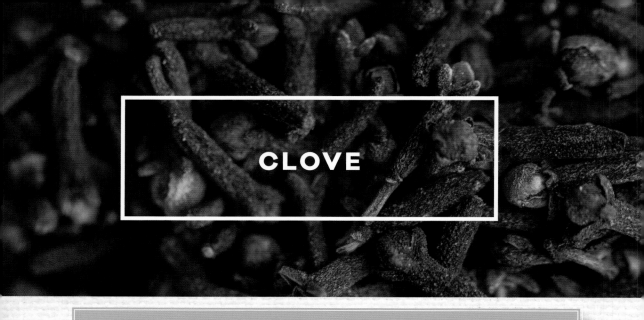

CLOVE

BOTANICAL NAME: *SYZYGIUM AROMATICUM*

In ancient China, courtiers at the Han court held cloves in their mouths to freshen their breath before they had an audience with the emperor. Today, cloves are still used to sweeten breath. Modern dental preparations numb tooth and gum pain and quell infection with clove essential oil or its main constituent, eugenol. Simply inhaling the fragrance was once said to improve eyesight and fend off the plague. Clove's scent developed a reputation, now backed by science, for being stimulating. The fragrance was also believed to be an aphrodisiac. Cloves were so valuable that a Frenchman risked his life to steal a clove tree from the Dutch colonies in Indonesia and plant it in French ground. Once established, the slender evergreen trees bear buds for at least a century.

The familiar clove buds used to poke hams and flavor mulled wine are picked while still unripe and dried before being shipped or distilled into essential oil.

As an antiseptic and pain reliever, clove essential oil relieves toothaches, flu, colds, and bronchial congestion. The essential oil irritates skin and mucous membranes, however, so be sure to dilute it before use. In a heating liniment, clove essential oil helps sore muscles and arthritis. Mix 30 drops of clove essential oil in one ounce of apple cider vinegar, shake well, and dab on athlete's foot. The oil is remarkably effective at curbing mold problems in bathrooms and other damp places.

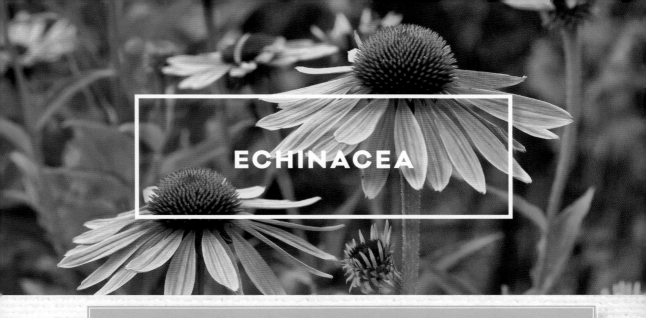

ECHINACEA

BOTANICAL NAME: *ECHINACEA PURPUREA*

Also known as the purple coneflower, this showy perennial was used by the Native Americans and adopted by the early settlers as a medicine. Members of the medical profession in early America relied heavily on echinacea, but it fell from favor with the advent of pharmaceutical medicine and antibiotics. Physicians have subsequently rediscovered the benefits of echinacea. Many forms of echinacea are available to choose from; Germany has registered more than 40 different echinacea products.

Long used for infectious diseases and poor immune function, echinacea extractions are also used today to help treat cancer, chronic fatigue syndrome, and AIDS. Research has shown echinacea stimulates the body's natural immune function. It also increases both the number and the activity of white blood cells, raises the level of interferon, and stimulates blood cells to engulf invading microbes. Echinacea also increases the production of substances the body produces naturally to fight cancers and disease. It contains enzymes that destroy bacterial enzymes. This gentle plant is completely innocuous—it can be used safely by children and the elderly.

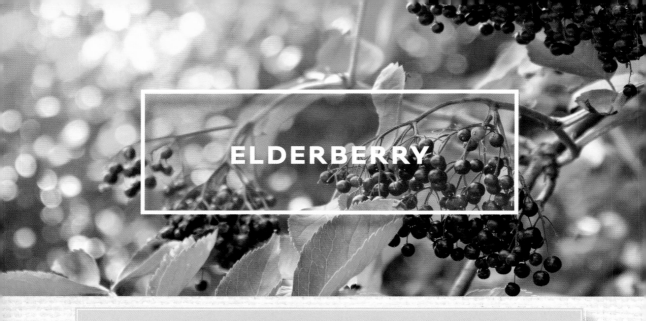

ELDERBERRY

BOTANICAL NAME: *SAMBUCUS NIGRA*

Elderberry has probably been used medicinally and nutritively for as long as human beings have gathered plants. In the kitchen, the berries are used to make jams, jellies, chutneys, preserves, wines, and teas. For decades, elder flower water was on the dressing tables of proper young ladies who used it to treat sunburn and eradicate freckles. It is still sometimes used in Europe for these purposes. Yellow and violet dyes are made from the leaves and berries, respectively. Elderberry has been used as a mild digestive stimulant and diaphoretic. Elder flowers decrease inflammation so are often included in preparations to treat burns and swellings and in cosmetics that reduce puffiness.

The berries have been used traditionally in Europe to treat flu, gout, and rheumatism as well as to improve general health. Several tales attribute longevity to the elderberry. Recent studies in Israel found the berry is a potent antiviral that fights influenza virus B, the cause of one of the common forms of flu. Recognizing that it has long been used as a flu remedy, researchers at the Hebrew University Hadasah Medical Centre in Jerusalem conducted clinical studies and found the berry reduced fever, coughs, and muscle pain within 24 hours. After taking an elderberry syrup only two days, almost two-thirds of those with influenza reported complete recovery. The Centre also found that elderberry stimulates the immune system.

The berries are currently under investigation for their ability to inhibit the herpes and Epstein-Barr viruses as well as HIV, the virus that causes AIDS. The berries are rich in compounds that improve heart and circulatory health.

The raw fruit contains a chemical that produces cyanide. The berries must be cooked before use. Eating raw elderberries may cause nausea and vomiting, and more serious effects at high doses.

Elderberry Products

Commercial elderberry preparations are plentiful (even more so in Europe), and include lozenges, capsules, tinctures, syrups, and extracts—as well as the dried berries themselves, which can be brewed into a tea. There is no standard dose or method of use, so a little personal experimentation is called for. You can even make your own elderberry jelly.

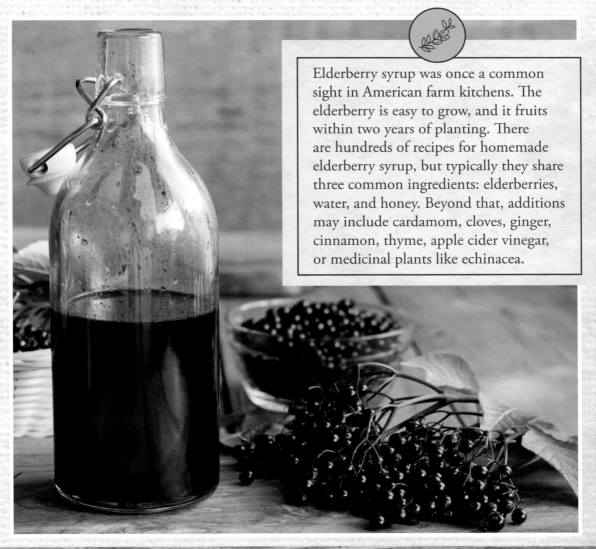

Elderberry syrup was once a common sight in American farm kitchens. The elderberry is easy to grow, and it fruits within two years of planting. There are hundreds of recipes for homemade elderberry syrup, but typically they share three common ingredients: elderberries, water, and honey. Beyond that, additions may include cardamom, cloves, ginger, cinnamon, thyme, apple cider vinegar, or medicinal plants like echinacea.

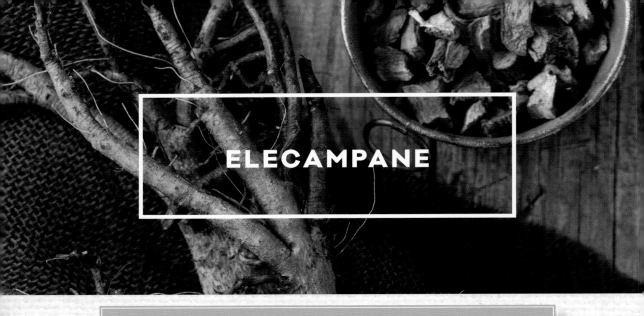

ELECAMPANE

BOTANICAL NAME: *INULA HELENIUM*

Elecampane's Latin name, *helenium*, refers to the legend that Helen of Troy carried a handful of elecampane on the day Paris abducted her, sparking the Trojan War. Perhaps she carried it because she had worms: Elecampane has been used for centuries to expel parasites in the digestive system, and today we know it contains at least one compound that expels intestinal worms (alantolactone). But elecampane has been used most often for treating respiratory diseases. It is especially good for shortness of breath and bronchial problems. Early American colonists grew it for use as an expectorant; in Europe, people with asthma chewed on the root. Indian Ayurvedic physicians prescribe elecampane for chest conditions. In China, the plant is used to make syrup, lozenges, and candy to treat bronchitis and asthma.

European studies show that elecampane promotes menstruation and may be useful in reducing blood pressure. The herb also has been shown to have some sedative effect. The root is added to many medicines and used as a flavoring for sweets. Cordials and sugar cakes are still made from it in parts of Europe.

Avoid elecampane if you're pregnant, as the herb has been used traditionally to promote menstruation. Studies have shown that a small dose of elecampane lowers blood sugar levels in animals, but higher doses raise them. Thus, people with diabetes should be careful when using the herb.

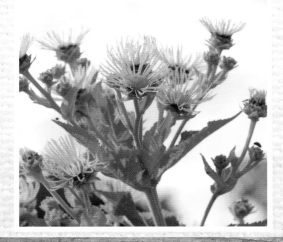

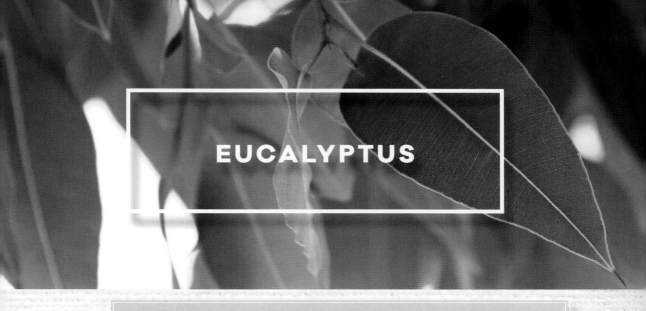

EUCALYPTUS

Eucalyptus or "gum" trees originated in Australia and Tasmania, but they are now found in subtropical regions all over the globe. Eucalyptus' thick, long, bluish-green leaves are distilled to provide essential oil. Blue gum eucalyptus, the most widely cultivated variety, provides most of the commercially available oil, although with more than 600 species, there are a variety of scents. Aromatherapists sometimes favor the more relaxing qualities and pleasant scent of the lemony *E. citriodora*. A very inexpensive oil, eucalyptus is used liberally to scent aftershaves, deodorants, and colognes, and as an antiseptic in mouthwashes and household cleansers.

Eucalyptus is an all-purpose topical remedy. It is antibacterial, antiviral, and antiseptic. Especially appropriate for skin eruptions and oily complexions, it is also used for acne, herpes, and chicken pox. For a homemade preparation, mix eucalyptus essential oil with an equal amount of apple cider vinegar and dab on problem areas. This mix can also be used as an antiseptic on wounds, boils, and insect bites.

It is the most popular essential oil steam for relieving sinus and lung congestion such as asthma. Inhale the steam, add one or two drops of oil to a compress, or put three or four drops in your bath. As a liniment it relieves rheumatic, arthritic, and other types of pain.

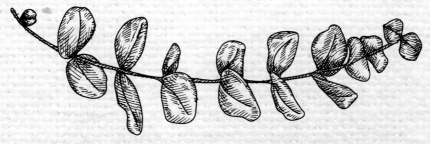

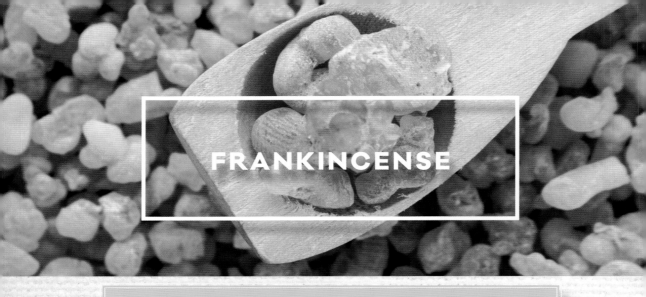

FRANKINCENSE

BOTANICAL NAME: *BOSWELLIA*

Frankincense comes from a variety of trees known as *Boswellia*. The frankincense burned as church incense today is the same as that used by ancient peoples who inhabited the Middle East and North Africa. Eventually the use of frankincense spread throughout Europe and eastward into India, and it was burned as an offering to the gods of many cultures.

Its antiseptic and skin-healing properties fight bacterial and fungal skin infections and boils. Although it can be expensive, only a little of the essential oil is needed at a time. For problem skin areas, just a few drops of frankincense oil diluted in an equal amount of carrier oil are needed. Frankincense is excellent on mature skin and acne. It can even help fade unsightly scars. It is especially good when middle-aged women experience those conditions and also want to prevent wrinkles. Make a compress or massage oil with frankincense for breast cysts or for infection of the lungs, reproductive organs, or urinary tract.

As an antiseptic, the oil can be added to homemade disinfecting sprays to help eliminate airborne bacteria and viruses.

Frankincense originates as a fragrant tree resin. Once the resin has hardened, it is harvested. The resulting pieces are known as frankincense tears.

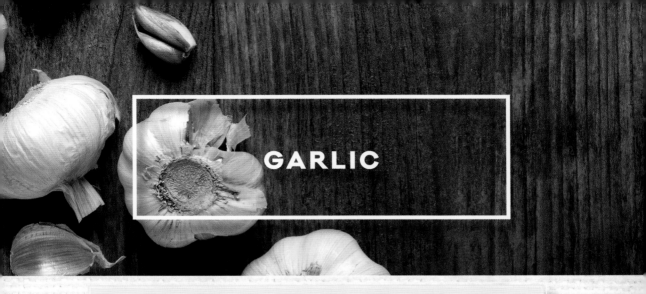

GARLIC

BOTANICAL NAME: *ALLIUM SATIVUM*

The wonders of garlic have been with us for millennia. Writings from ancient Egypt, Greece, India, and China all make mention of the humble garlic clove. It has long been used in many cultures to improve health or transform meals into delicious, aromatic delights. Its ability to enhance flavor is undeniable, while the extent of its healing benefits continues to be revealed. In many historic cultures, garlic was used medicinally but not in cooking. That might surprise us today, but were our ancestors able to travel into the future to visit us, they would likely think us rather dense for our culture's general lack of appreciation for the bulb's healing qualities.

Traditionally, garlic bulbs were prepared in a variety of ways for medicinal purposes. The juice of the bulb might be extracted and taken internally for one purpose, while the bulb might be ground into a paste for external treatment of other health problems. In the minds of the superstitious, simply possessing garlic was enough to bring good luck and protect against evil or mysterious entities.

Garlic played its first starring role in modern medical treatment during World War I. The Russians used garlic on the front lines to treat battle wounds and fight infection, and medics used moss that was soaked in garlic as an antiseptic to pack wounds. In the first part of the 20th century, garlic saw plenty of action off the battlefield, too. Even though penicillin was discovered in 1928, the demand for it among the general population often outstripped the supply, so many people continued with the treatments they had used with some success before, including garlic.

The pungent, ancient remedy has found its way to modern times. Herbalists have long touted garlic for a number of health problems, from preventing colds and treating intestinal problems to lowering blood cholesterol and reducing heart disease risk. Garlic remedies abound—and scientific research has begun to support the usefulness of some of them. Garlic's popularity today is due in part to the efforts of scientists around the world. They have identified a number of sulfur-containing compounds in garlic that have important medicinal properties.

Potent Medicinal Compounds

If you were to look at or sniff an intact garlic clove sitting on a cutting board, you'd never suspect the potent aroma and healing properties within. Whack it with a knife, however, and you open a portal!

Cutting, crushing, or chewing a garlic clove activates numerous sulfurous substances. When these substances come into contact with oxygen, they form compounds that have therapeutic properties. The most researched, and possibly the most medicinally powerful, of these potent compounds are allicin and ajoene.

One of the difficulties in comparing studies of garlic's effectiveness in humans is that there are many different forms of garlic used in the studies. One may contain more of an active ingredient than another. For example:

Fresh cloves of garlic—chopped or chewed: These may impart the highest amount of allicin, but they have not been well studied yet.

Fresh cloves of garlic—swallowed whole: These showed no therapeutic value in a limited number of studies that have been done.

Dehydrated garlic powder—made into tablets or capsules: This form often provided some therapeutic value, but allicin content of these products varies within and among brands.

Enteric-coated garlic tablets: These are treated so they do not dissolve until they reach your intestines, rather than your stomach. Some studies show that enteric-coated tablets don't dissolve soon enough to release the allicin they contain. This type of tablet usually prevents garlic odor on the breath.

Nonenteric-coated garlic tablets: Tablets effective in studies were standardized to contain 1.3 percent allicin. These may be more effective than the enteric-coated tablets, but they do cause garlic breath.

Aged garlic extract: One of the active compounds in this form is ajoene. There have been conflicting results in studies of health benefits.

Garlic oil: Shows little therapeutic value in studies.

Garlic's Attack on Plaque

Garlic contains several powerful antioxidants—compounds that prevent oxidation, a harmful process in the body. One of them is selenium, a mineral that is a component of glutathione peroxidase, a powerful antioxidant that the body makes to defend itself. Glutathione peroxidase works with vitamin E to form a superantioxidant defense system.

Other antioxidants in garlic include vitamin C, which helps reduce the damage that LDL cholesterol can cause, and quercetin, a phytochemical. (Phytochemicals are chemical substances found in plants that may have health benefits for people.) Garlic also has trace amounts of the mineral manganese, which is an important component of an antioxidant enzyme called superoxide dismutase.

Oxidation

Oxidation is related to oxygen, a vital element to every aspect of our lives, so why is oxidation so harmful? Think about when rust accumulates on your car or garden tools and eventually destroys the metal. That rust is an example of oxidation. Similarly, when your body breaks down glucose for energy, free radicals are produced. These free radicals start oxidizing—and damaging—cellular tissue. It's as if your bloodstream and blood vessels are "rusting out."

Antioxidants destroy free radicals, including those that are products of environmental factors, such as ultraviolet rays, air pollutants, cigarette smoke, rancid oils, and pesticides. The body keeps a steady supply of antioxidants ready to neutralize free radicals. Unfortunately, sometimes the number of free radicals can overwhelm the body's antioxidant stock, especially if we're not getting enough of the antioxidant nutrients. When free radicals harm the cells that line your arteries, your body tries to mend the damage by producing a sticky spackle-like substance. However, as mentioned earlier, this substance attracts cholesterol and debris that build up within the arteries, causing progressive plaque formation. The more plaque in your arteries, the more your health is in danger.

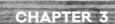

Infection Fighter

Garlic's potential to combat heart disease has received a lot of attention, but it should get just as much for its antimicrobial properties. Raw garlic has proven itself since ancient times as an effective killer of bacteria and viruses. Once again, we can thank allicin.

Laboratory studies confirm that raw garlic has antibacterial and antiviral properties. Not only does it knock out many common cold and flu viruses but its effectiveness also spans a broad range of both gram-positive and gram-negative bacteria, fungus, intestinal parasites, and yeast. Cooking garlic, however, destroys the allicin, so you'll need to use raw garlic to prevent or fight infections.

One excellent demonstration of garlic's antibacterial power can be found in a study conducted at the University of California, Irvine. Garlic juice was tested against a wide spectrum of potential pathogens, including several known antibiotic-resistant strains of bacteria. It showed significant activity against the pathogens. Even more exciting was the fact that garlic juice still retained significant antimicrobial activity even in dilutions ranging up to 1:128 of the original juice.

Eating raw garlic may help combat the pathogens that attack our bodies. It has been used internally as a remedy for years, but now the plant is being put to the test scientifically for such uses. So far, its grades are quite good as researchers pit it against a variety of bacteria.

For eons, herbalists loaded soups and other foods with garlic and placed garlic compresses on people's chests to provide relief from colds and chest congestion. Now the Mayo Clinic has stated, "preliminary reports suggest that garlic may reduce the severity of upper respiratory tract infection."

A study published in the July/August 2001 issue of *Advances in Therapy* examined the stinking rose's ability to fight the common cold. The study involved 146 volunteers divided into two groups. One group took a garlic supplement for 12 weeks during the winter months, while the other group received a placebo. The group that received garlic had significantly fewer colds—and the colds that they did get went away faster—than the placebo group.

Finally, in the January 2005 issue of *Antimicrobial Agents and Chemotherapy*, researchers reported the results of an investigation into whether fresh garlic extract would inhibit *C. albicans*, a cause of yeast infections. The extract was very effective in the first hour of exposure to *C. albicans*, but the effectiveness decreased during the 48-hour period it was measured. However, traditional antifungal medications also have the same declining effectiveness as time passes.

External Treatment

Applying a topical solution of raw garlic and water may stop wounds from getting infected. (Simply crush one clove of garlic and mix it with one-third of a cup of clean water. Use the solution within three hours because it will lose its potency over time.) A garlic solution used as a footbath several times a day is traditionally believed to improve athlete's foot.

Using garlic oil extract appears to work better than the old folk remedy of tying or taping a slice of garlic to a wart. If the slice of garlic is bigger than the wart or moves just a bit, it blisters the healthy surrounding skin (of course, you have the same risk when using wart-removing products that contain acid). Garlic's phytochemical compounds are strong enough to create chemical burns, so always apply externally with caution and do not use on young children. One way you can protect the surrounding healthy skin is to smear petroleum jelly on it before you apply the garlic.

Cancer Crusader

Some scientists think garlic may be able to help prevent one of the most dreaded maladies—cancer. The Mayo Clinic has reported that some studies using cancer cells in the laboratory, as well as some studies with animals and people, have suggested that eating garlic, especially unprocessed garlic, might reduce the risk of stomach and colon cancers. The National Institutes of Health's National Cancer Institute drew similar conclusions after reviewing 37 studies involving garlic and sulfur-containing compounds. Twenty-eight of those studies indicated garlic possessed at least some anticancer activity, especially toward prostate and stomach cancer.

Because the studies in question were merely observational, more studies are needed. Still, the research the National Cancer Institute reviewed found that it may not take much garlic to reap these anticancer benefits. Eating as few as two servings of garlic a week might be enough to help protect against colon cancer.

What gives garlic this wonderful gift? Several factors, including antioxidants and those same sulfur-containing agents we've discussed before, including allicin. Allicin appears to protect colon cells from the toxic effects of cancer-causing agents. For instance, when meat is cooked with garlic, the herb reduces the production of cancer-causing compounds that would otherwise form when meat is grilled at high temperatures.

Garlic's potential ability to decrease *H. pylori* bacteria in the stomach may help prevent gastritis (inflammation of the stomach lining) from eventually evolving into cancer. (*H. pylori* is most famous for its link to stomach ulcers, but it can also cause chronic gastritis.) Numerous studies around the world indicate that garlic's sulfur-containing compounds have the potential to help prevent stomach cancer.

What Can't Garlic Cure?

Sore throats: This Amish remedy works well—if you can stand it. Peel a fresh clove, slice it in half, and place 1 piece in each cheek. Suck on the garlic like a cough drop. Occasionally, crush your teeth against the garlic, not to bite it in half, but to release its allicin, a chemical that can kill the bacteria that causes strep.

Laxative: In the raw, garlic has a laxative effect for many. Eat it mixed with onion, raw or cooked, and with milk or yogurt for best results.

Coughs: Along with its antibiotic and antiviral properties, garlic is also an expectorant—so it helps you cough up the stubborn bacteria and/or mucus that are languishing in your lungs. A cup of garlic broth may do the trick, and it is easy to prepare. Smash 1 to 3 cloves garlic (or more, depending on how strong you like your garlic), add 2 quarts water, and boil on low heat for one hour. Strain and sip slowly.

Diverticulosis: This can help prevent infection: Eat 1 clove, three times a day. Chop it into a salad or add it to soup or stew. Pasta sauce, however, is not a good choice since tomato-based, spicy, and acidic foods can exacerbate symptoms.

Yeast infection: Eating 2 fresh garlic cloves a day, either plain or minced and tossed in a salad or sauce, may prevent yeast infections or help clear up a case of thrush.

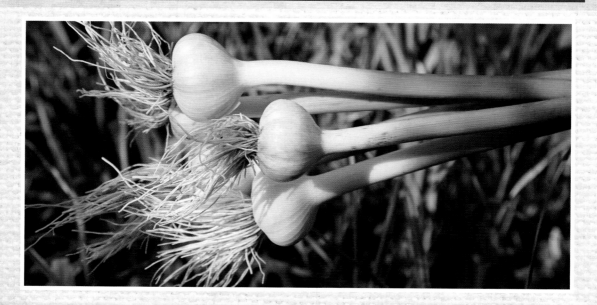

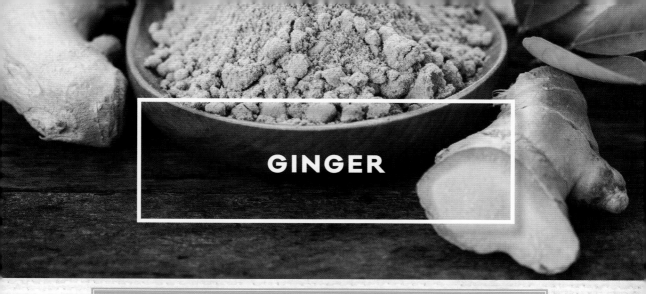

GINGER

BOTANICAL NAME: *ZINGIBER OFFICINALE*

Ginger ale, gingerbread, gingersnaps . . . we're familiar with commercial ginger products from childhood on, but ginger has a lot more going for it than just a flavorful food additive. This botanical and popular spice is native to southeast Asia. Fresh ginger root is a staple in Asian cooking. Dried and powdered, it's used in medicine. Ginger is high in volatile essential oils. Ginger root powder may be useful in improving pain, stiffness, lack of mobility, and swelling. Larger dosages in the area of 3 or 4 grams of ginger powder daily appear most effective. But powder may not be the only effective form of ginger root—one study demonstrated benefits from the ingestion of lightly cooked ginger.

Ginger has a long history of use as a general tonic and remedy for forms of nausea like morning sickness, motion sickness, and nausea accompanying gastroenteritis (more commonly called stomach flu). As a stomach calming aid,

ginger also reduces gas, bloating, and indigestion, and aids in the absorption and the body's use of other nutrients and medicines. It is also a valuable deterrent to intestinal worms, particularly roundworms. Ginger may even improve some cases of constant severe dizziness and vertigo. It may be both a therapy and a preventive treatment for some migraine headaches. Ginger also prevents platelets from clumping together in the bloodstream. This serves to thin the blood and reduce the risk of atherosclerosis and blood clots.

Ginger is a potent expectorant that works well in tea. Steep a half teaspoon ginger, a pinch of ground cloves, and a pinch of cinnamon in one cup of boiling water to ease bronchitis and other respiratory ailments. A strong ginger-based beverage can also help break a high fever.

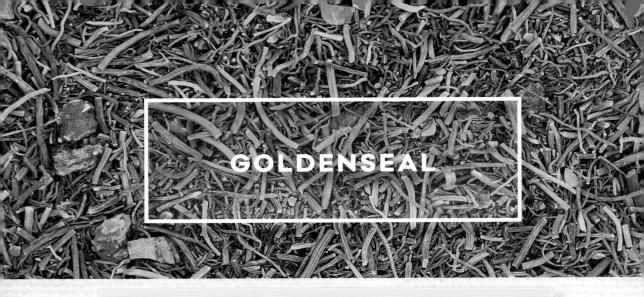

GOLDENSEAL

BOTANICAL NAME: *HYDRASTIS CANADENSIS*

The Cherokee Indians mixed powdered goldenseal root with bear grease and slathered their bodies to protect themselves from mosquitoes and other insects. Pioneers adopted the herb and used it to treat wounds, rashes, mouth sores, morning sickness, liver and stomach complaints, internal hemorrhaging, depressed appetite, constipation, and urinary and uterine problems.

One of goldenseal's active ingredients is hydrastine, which affects circulation, muscle tone, and uterine contractions. The herb is also an antiseptic, astringent, and antibiotic, making it effective for treating eye and other types of infections. Berberine and related alkaloids have been credited with goldenseal's antimicrobial effects. Goldenseal makes a good antiseptic skin wash for wounds and for internal skin surfaces, such as in the vagina and ear; it also treats canker sores and infected gums. The herb has been found to fight a number of disease-causing microbes, including *Staphylococcus* and *Streptococcus* organisms

Berberine may be responsible for increasing white blood cell activity and promoting blood flow in the liver and spleen. Berberine has been used in China to combat the reduction of white blood cells that commonly follows chemotherapy and radiation treatment for cancer. Studies suggest it may have potential in the treatment of brain and skin cancers.

Hydrastine accumulates in the system and is toxic in large doses. Berberine may lower blood pressure, but hydrastine raises it, so avoid the herb if you have high blood pressure, heart disease, or glaucoma.

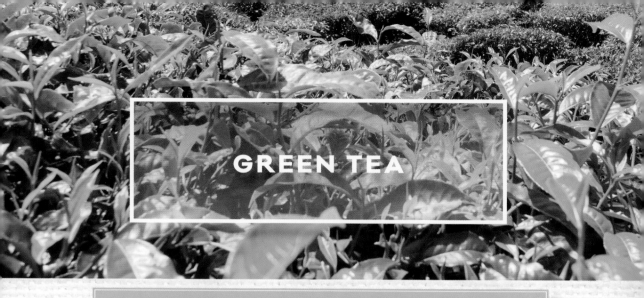

GREEN TEA

BOTANICAL NAME: *CAMELLIA SINENSIS*

"Better to be deprived of food for three days, than tea for one," goes the old Chinese proverb. The medicinal power of tea has been recognized in eastern Asia for thousands of years. It is one of the most widely consumed beverages in the world. It has been traditionally claimed to help with digestion, enhance concentration, assist with bowel movements, relieve headaches, assist with weight loss, and contribute to longevity. Modern studies of green tea's constituents bear out the traditional wisdom. Green tea does it all.

Green tea provides broad antimicrobial action—it is effective against *E. coli, Proteus vulgaris, Pseudomonas fluorescens, Salmonella,* and *Staphylococcus aureus.* The catechins in green tea inhibit the ulcer-causing *H. pylori.* And amazingly, green tea extract seems to reverse the antibiotic resistance of some bacteria.

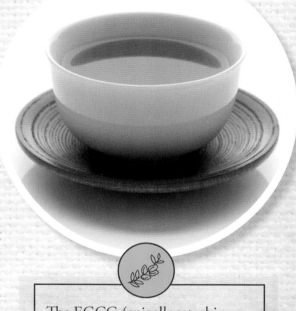

The EGCG (epigallocatechin gallate) in a simply-prepared cup of green tea is effective against certain mouth bacteria.

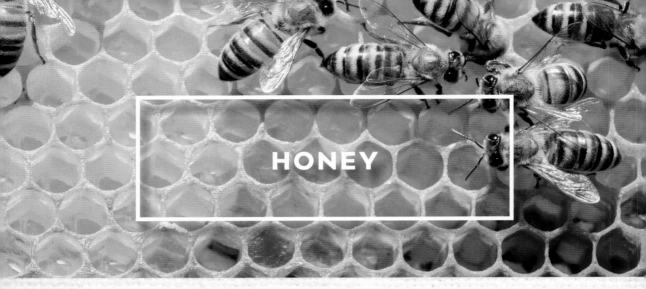

HONEY

Honey is a unique substance, and the only one in this book created by insects. Bees create honey to provide their colonies with food. First a bee gathers floral nectar and then mixes it with special proteins and enzymes that converts the honey into glucose and fructose. A small amount of the glucose is modified by another enzyme and converted to gluconic acid and hydrogen peroxide. This provides protection from bacteria, mold, fungi, and other microbes. The honey is then deposited in the beeswax comb. Bees in the hive reduce the moisture of the honey by fanning their wings. Once this is done, the bees cap the honeycomb with wax. Simple-sounding, but the resulting substance has near-miraculous healing properties.

Nectar from flowers provides the raw material that honey is made from.

All-purpose Panacea

Honey is the only food that includes all the nutrients necessary to sustain life. Honey and bee pollen contain water, as well as all 22 minerals and enzymes that the human body needs. As an antimicrobial, its full scope of action is still not fully understood. It has now been proven that honey will inhibit pathogens like *E. coli*, salmonella, and the pernicious hospital bugs *Staphylococcus aureus* and *Pseudomonas aeruginosa*. Studies have also shown that it is a more effective nighttime cough suppressant than some over-the-counter cough remedies. Honey-based dressings are now routinely used by healthcare professionals to treat infected skin wounds.

Help that sore throat—and promote the flow of mucus—by drinking a cup of hot tea mixed with 1 tablespoon of honey and 2 drops of lemon juice. This even works with plain hot water instead of tea. These are good tonics to help ease laryngitis, as well. More throat relief comes when honey soothes and vinegar kills bacteria. Whip up a batch of homemade cough syrup by mixing 1/4 cup each of apple cider vinegar and honey. Pour into a bottle or jar that can be sealed tightly. Take 1 tablespoon every 4 hours, shaking well before each dose. Sore throats also respond well to this drink: In a glass of water, mix 1 teaspoon of honey, 3 tablespoons of lime juice, and 1 tablespoon of pineapple juice. Sip to obtain soothing relief.

For digestive maladies and upset stomach, try this: a teaspoon or two of honey mixed with milk. The mixture works well either warm or cold, but some people swear by warm milk. You may also prevent indigestion by taking a spoonful of honey sprinkled with a bit of cinnamon before beginning a meal. Honey taken by itself or mixed with water, milk, or tea can remedy feelings of nausea too.

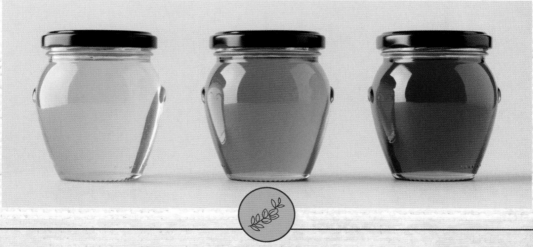

General note: When shopping for honey, you'll see that some kinds are lighter than others. In general, the darker the honey is, the higher its antimicrobial potential.

Manuka Honey

Manuka honey is made by Australia and New Zealand bees that frequent the manuka bush. Manuka is reputedly a more powerful antimicrobial than other types of honey. While this is partially due to the high concentration of the powerful antimicrobial methylglyoxal found in this honey, it has been shown that even after this compound is neutralized, manuka still displays high bactericidal activity. Thus far, this honey has been shown to have an inhibitory effect on 60 species of bacteria. It is generally used for treating minor wounds and burns. It is also considered effective for eye, ear, and sinus infections, helping to reduce inflammation in the body, treating gastrointestinal problems, and treating cancer.

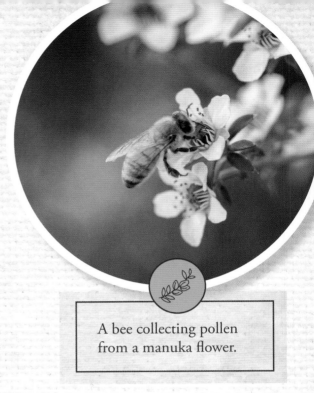

A bee collecting pollen from a manuka flower.

Propolis

Along with nectar, bees collect gummy, resinous substances from the bark of trees and from buds and carry them back to the hive in tiny baskets on their feet. This raw material is turned into propolis, a viscous substance the bees use to plug cracks and varnish the interior of the hive. Propolis has strong disinfectant properties. Ancient cultures understood its benefits and used it to treat skin afflictions like boils, ulcers, and abscesses. Propolis is active against all four classes of pathogens, but it is especially effective against bacteria. For infections of the mouth, throat, and upper respiratory tract, you can chew a propolis paste or fragments slowly, to keep the active compounds in contact with the site of the infection. Propolis is also found in creams and ointments and used topically for skin disorders.

Propolis in its raw form.

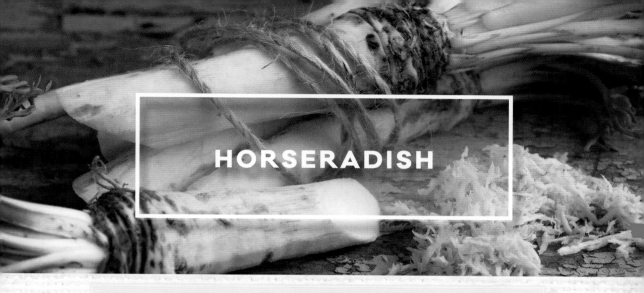

HORSERADISH

BOTANICAL NAME: *ARMORIACIA RUSTICANA*

Have you ever bitten into a roast beef sandwich and thought your nose was on fire? The sandwich probably contained horseradish. Even a tiny taste of this potent condiment seems to go straight to your nose. Whether on a sandwich or in an herbal preparation, horseradish clears sinuses, increases facial circulation, and promotes expulsion of mucus. Horseradish is helpful for sinus infections because it encourages your body to get rid of mucus. One way a sinus infection starts is with the accumulation of thick mucus in the sinuses: Stagnant mucus is the perfect breeding ground for bacteria to multiply and cause a painful infection. Horseradish can help thin and move out older, thicker mucus accumulations. If you are prone to developing sinus infections, try taking horseradish the minute you feel a cold coming on. Herbalists also recommend horseradish for common colds, influenza, and lung congestion. Incidentally, don't view the increase of mucus production after horseradish therapy as a sign your cold is worsening. The free-flowing mucus is a positive sign that your body is ridding itself of wastes. Horseradish has a mild natural antibiotic effect and it will stimulate urine production. Thus it has also been used for urinary infections. Horseradish can make an effective heat-producing poultice that alleviates the pain of arthritis and neuralgia.

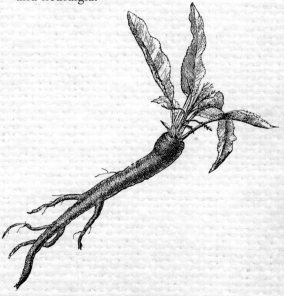

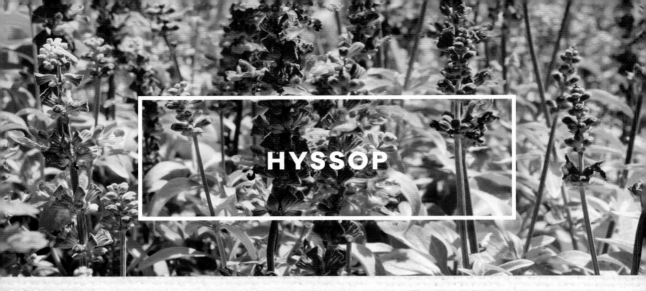

HYSSOP

BOTANICAL NAME: *HYSSOPUS OFFICINALIS*

Hyssop is native to southern Europe and the Middle East, and has been used medicinally since antiquity due to its antiseptic, cough-relieving, and expectorant properties. It was used in the Middle Ages as a pest repellant and to ward off bad smells and even the plague. Hyssop baths were once used in England to treat rheumatism. It has a bright medicinal smell that many people will associate with mouthwash.

Hyssop has been shown to prevent infections when applied to wounds, and is effective against viral infections such as colds and flu. In laboratory tests, it destroys herpesvirus. Its antispasmodic properties make it a great choice for calming coughs, and hyssop tea can soothe a sore throat. When used in steam inhalation, the oil helps to ease breathing and clear the respiratory tract.

Hyssop Essential Oil

The essential oil is a particularly effective antimicrobial. To treat minor skin wounds, mix a few drops of the oil with a carrier oil and apply to the affected area. As an antibacterial agent, it makes a great addition to acne-fighting cleansers. Its astringent properties help tone the skin.

Hyssop is a great addition to your home-cleaning arsenal. Simply diffuse the oil to help rid the air of pathogens. Add it to kitchen and bathroom cleaners to help disinfect countertops and other surfaces.

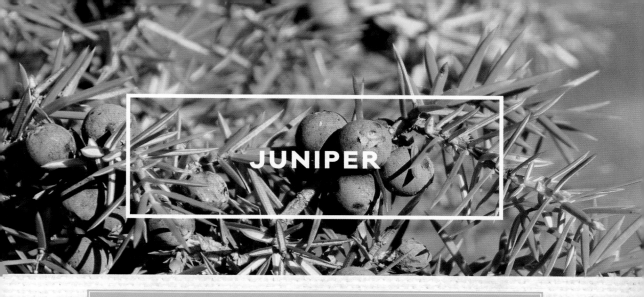

JUNIPER

BOTANICAL NAME: *JUNIPERUS COMMUNIS*

Medicinal use of juniper in recorded history goes back to an Egyptian papyrus (circa 1500 BC) containing a formula to cure tapeworms. Burning juniper branches was found to ward off contagious diseases, so medieval physicians chewed the berries while on duty and burned the branches in hospitals. Modern herbalists still consider chewing berries a useful way to ward off airborne viruses when one is exposed to sick people. In World War II, the French returned to burning juniper in hospitals as an antiseptic when their supply of drugs ran low. The most potent oil is distilled from the berries. The oil is an excellent addition to disinfecting room sprays.

Juniper berries contain nearly 90 chemical compounds. They are high in flavonoids and polyphenols. Antioxidant phytochemicals include alpha-pinene, cadinene, limonene, myrcene, borneol, caryophyllene and germacrene. Thanks to this abundant antioxidant content, the oil has a host of healing applications. The astringent juniper is antiseptic, antibacterial, antifungal, and antiviral. It is most commonly added to massage oils, liniments, and baths to treat soreness, arthritic and rheumatic pain, varicose veins, and hemorrhoids. Used in steam inhalations, it relieves bronchial congestion, infection, and bronchial spasms. In tea form, juniper berry has a diuretic effect. This, combined with its antimicrobial, cleansing action, makes it a remedy for treating urinary tract infections.

Cosmetically it is suitable for treating acne and eczema conditions. The essential oil's fresh scent and odor-killing effects make it a great addition to natural deodorants.

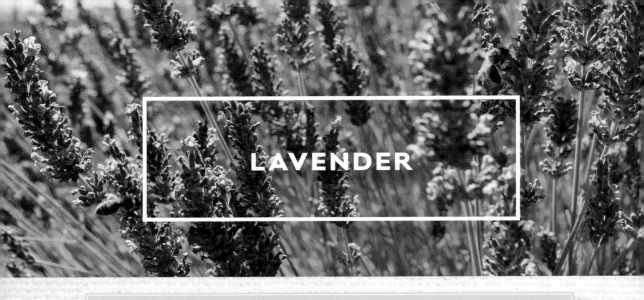

LAVENDER

BOTANICAL NAME: *LAVANDULA ANGUSTIFOLIA*

A well-loved Mediterranean herb, lavender has been associated with cleanliness since Romans first added it to their bathwater. In fact, the name comes from the Latin *lavandus*, meaning to wash. Today lavender remains a favorite for scenting clothing and closets, soaps, and even furniture polish. Lavender was traditionally inhaled to ease exhaustion, insomnia, irritability, and depression. Two related plants called spike (*L. latifolia*) and lavandin (*L. intermedia*) are produced in greater quantities; but they are more camphorous and harsher in scent, with inferior healing properties, although they are useful for disinfecting.

Lavender is among the safest and most widely used of all the aroma-therapy oils. It relieves muscle pain, migraines and other headaches, and inflammation. It is also one of the most antiseptic essential oils, treating many types of infection, including lung, sinus, and vaginal infections. Lavender is suitable for all skin types. Cosmetically, it appears to be a cell regenerator. It prevents scarring and stretch marks and reputedly slows the development of wrinkles. It is used on burns, sun-damaged skin, wounds, rashes, and, of course, skin infections.

Lavender essential oil is a classic broad-spectrum compound that can used against bacteria, fungi, parasites, and viruses. There are more powerful antibiotic essential oils, but lavender has the benefit of being gentle enough to use on the skin.

Healing and Relaxing

The multiple benefits and applications of lavender essential oil make it a very special plant. Along with its disinfectant and antibiotic properties, lavender also has the ability to boost overall wellness. Lavender tea and powdered capsules are taken to treat anxiety, depression, insomnia, physical pain, and headaches. Whether taken internally, applied to the skin, or simply inhaled, lavender works as an anxiolytic (an anxiety reliever) and sedative. In one study, simply inhaling lavender essential oil was shown to significantly reduce the pain experienced during a migraine headache. Lavender's soothing effects on the nervous system appear to reduce blood pressure and heart rate. As an anti-inflammatory and analgesic it can significantly reduce joint and back pain.

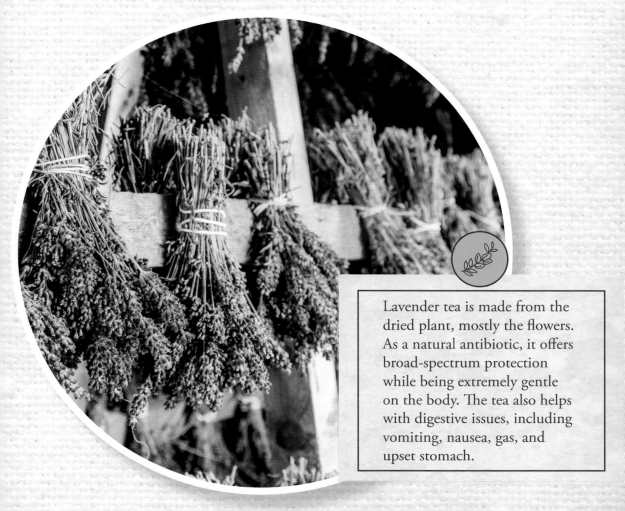

Lavender tea is made from the dried plant, mostly the flowers. As a natural antibiotic, it offers broad-spectrum protection while being extremely gentle on the body. The tea also helps with digestive issues, including vomiting, nausea, gas, and upset stomach.

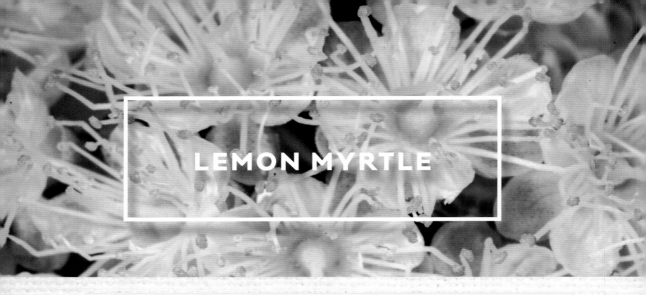

LEMON MYRTLE

BOTANICAL NAME: *BACKHOUSIA CITRIODORA*

Named after English botanist James Backhouse, *Backhousia citriodora* was once commonly known as lemon-scented myrtle. Eventually, the name was shortened to "lemon myrtle," to help the edible herb achieve more popularity in the culinary world. The lemony dried leaves are used in everything from sweet desserts to savory pastas, and are also popular in soaps, lotions, and bath products. The plant is native to Australia, where indigenous people have used it for medicine for hundreds of years due to its antimicrobial properties. Even today, the majority of lemon myrtle used for essential oil is grown only in Queensland and New South Wales, Australia.

Lemon myrtle's antimicrobial properties make it ideal for treating skin conditions such as acne and psoriasis, or preventing infections in minor cuts and scrapes. The essential oil can also ease itching and inflammation caused by insect bites and stings. It may help boost the immune system and keep colds and flu at bay. A few drops in bathwater help to relax the mind as well as the muscles. Lemon myrtle essential oil is an excellent addition to housecleaning products, thanks to its antiseptic qualities and uplifting scent.

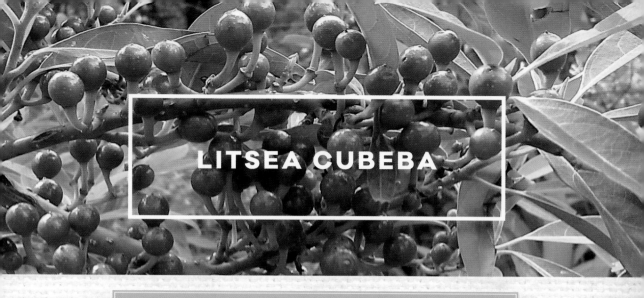

LITSEA CUBEBA

BOTANICAL NAME: *LITSEA CUBEBA*

Also known as aromatic litsea and may chang, litsea cubeba is an evergreen tree native to Southeast Asia. The tree bears a fruit that resembles a pepper, giving it the nickname "mountain pepper." The essential oil—which has a lemony, citrusy scent similar to lemongrass—is extracted from these ripened and dried pepper-like fruits. The oil has traditionally been used in Chinese medicine to help with digestive issues, muscle aches, and asthma, and to relieve stress and anxiety.

Effective in killing bacteria, viruses, and fungi, litsea cubeba aids a host of problems, including acne, athlete's foot, insect bites, and ringworm. The uplifting scent has been used for hundreds of years in aromatherapy to in-

duce feelings of calm and reduce stress. A few drops added to a carrier oil and massaged into your stomach can reduce indigestion and stomach upset. The oil is disinfectant and makes a great addition to home cleaning solutions.

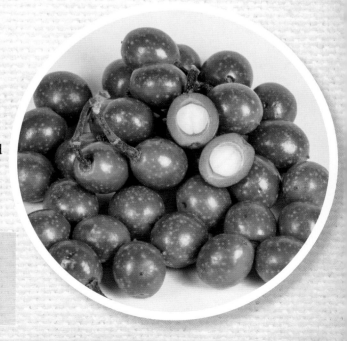

The fruits are ripened and dried before the essential oils are extracted.

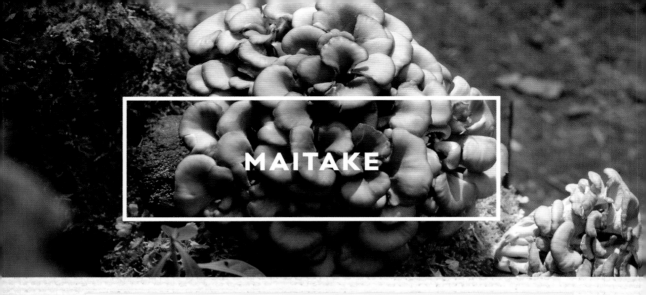

MAITAKE

BOTANICAL NAME: *GRIFOLA FRONDOSA*

Translating to "dancing mushroom" in Japanese, the maitake has been used in Japanese and Chinese medicine for thousands of years. It was said to have acquired its name when people would dance with glee upon finding it in the wild due to its tremendous healing properties. It has only gained popularity in North America over the last few decades. But that popularity now seems to be growing rapidly. Consumers are becoming aware of its immunity-boosting and anti-cancer properties. As if its potential to improve health is not enough, the maitake has the added benefit of tasting delicious. It is rich in many key nutrients and a staple of Japanese cooking.

Research is ongoing and, as with other mushroom varieties, there is a lack of hard scientific proof confirming the health benefits of the maitake. That said, many tests have indicated that those celebrating in the woods upon discovering this mushroom had ample reason to dance. The primary optimism seems to be in the areas of cancer treatment, blood pressure

and cholesterol control, as well as blood sugar regulation (diabetes).

The maitake mushroom has indicated an ability to suppress the growth of tumors in mice. At least one study of human cells was also promising in the area of cancer fighting. Maitake extract, taken in conjunction with a cancer-fighting protein, seemed to improve the effectiveness of the protein in killing human cancer cells. Other tests have produced a common theme: that the maitake mushroom might have the ability to slow, stop, or reverse the spread of cancer.

Cholesterol levels in mice were lowered after maitake extract was given in a 2013 experiment that also linked the mushroom to an increase in energy-boosting fatty acids. Its large supply of antioxidants also makes it one of many mushroom varieties thought to be key in controlling blood pressure. By keeping the arteries healthy, maitake might help lower the risk of heart disease and stroke in humans.

There is considerable laboratory evidence that maitake may help reduce inflammation, strengthen the immune system against any number of illnesses, and help control glucose levels in the blood. A 2014 study showed the mushroom may be hypoglycemic, lowering blood sugar and stopping the occurrence of insulin resistance—key success factors in the treatment of diabetes. Another study the following year indicated benefits to rats with type 2 diabetes.

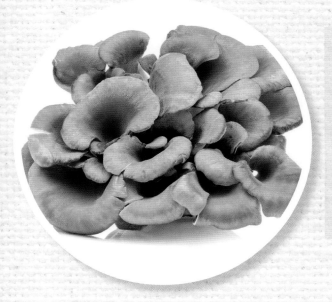

Native to parts of China, Japan, and North America, maitake mushrooms grow at the bottom of oak, elm, and maple trees. The Japanese varieties can grow to more than 50 pounds. The maitake has another nickname, "hen of the woods," because it can resemble a nesting hen's feathery tail.

While other medicinal mushrooms are typically taken in powder or liquid form as abstracts, maitake is popular in many recipes due to its taste. It is popular as a component of salads, stir-fries, in omelets, and even as a pizza topping.

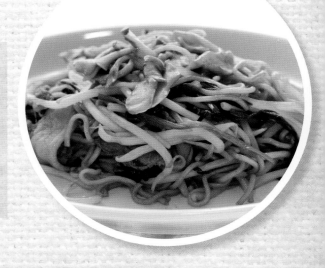

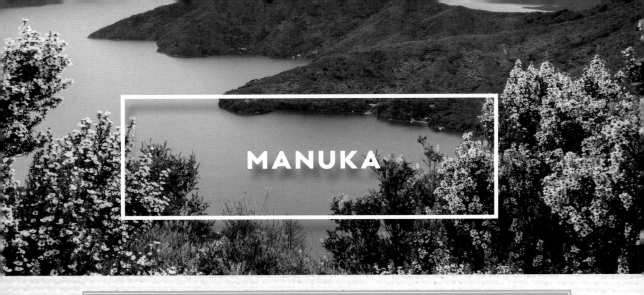

MANUKA

BOTANICAL NAME: *LEPTOSPERMUM SCOPARIUM*

Manuka honey may be getting most of the attention lately, but the essential oil of the manuka tree is another powerful natural antibiotic worthy of a place in everyone's medicine cabinet. The manuka is a small brushy tree native to Australia and New Zealand. It will grow in wet or dry locales and is famous for its ability to withstand drought. Small pink or white flowers bloom in summer or spring.

Manuka was dubbed "tea tree" by famed British explorer Captain James Cook. For this reason, it is still sometimes referred to that way. Captain Cook used the leaves of the manuka tree to brew tea (and also beer!), noting that the tea "has a very agreeable bitter scent and flavor when they are recent, but loses some of both when dried." Long before Captain Cook, the Maori in New Zealand were using manuka to cure fevers, treat colds, and soothe aching muscles. Today, manuka oil can be found in a myriad of skin care products on the market, but the pure essential oil is prized for a host of other benefits.

While manuka is related to the tea tree, the two species should not be confused. The oil distilled from manuka leaves is incredibly potent. Both manuka and tea tree oil can be used for many of the same purposes, but note: manuka essential oil is up to 30 times more effective against gram positive bacteria and up to 10 times more effective against fungi.

Manuka isn't just an antibacterial. Its anti-inflammatory properties help with a variety of skin conditions. It can diminish casual skin blemishes, scars, and stretch marks. It can drastically reduce the swelling, itching, and discomfort caused by insect bites and stings. It is effective against dandruff, psoriasis, and eczema. The oil promotes the development of new skin cells, making it an effective part of wound treatment. Mixed with aloe, it soothes burns and dry skin. Its antiviral properties help reduce the severity of cold sores. As an antifungal, it can be used to treat various strains of fungus, including athlete's foot, toenail fungus, and candida.

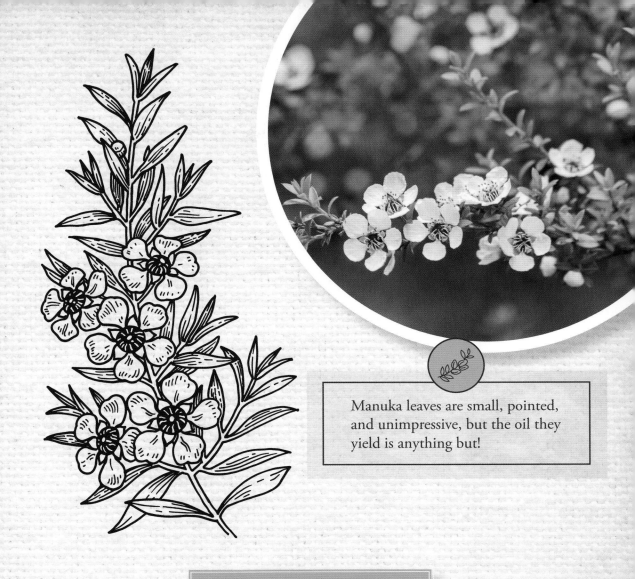

Manuka leaves are small, pointed, and unimpressive, but the oil they yield is anything but!

Cousin Kanuka

Related to Manuka and somewhat similar in appearance, Kanuka is endemic to New Zealand. The plant boasts many of the same benefits. The essential oil is becoming increasingly popular. It is a suitable substitute for tea tree oil for those looking for a more delicate scent. Typically, it is used topically to help with wound healing, to fight infection, reduce dandruff, and treat acne.

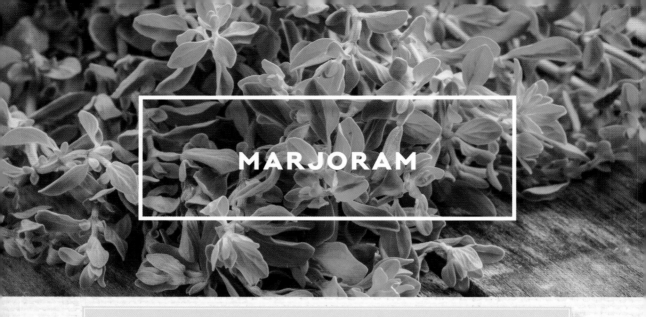

MARJORAM

BOTANICAL NAME: *ORIGANUM MARJORANA*

Marjoram is a bushy, spreading, perennial that produces small, oval leaves and knotlike shapes that blossom into tiny white or pink flowers from August through September. It is native to southwest Asia and has become naturalized in Mediterranean regions.

Traditionally, herbalists have prescribed marjoram to treat asthma, increase sweating, lower fevers, encourage menstruation, and, especially, relieve indigestion. European singers preserved their voices with marjoram tea sweetened with honey. Marjoram gargles and steam treatments relieve sinus congestion and hay fever. Its antioxidant properties are so potent they have been shown to be excellent food preservatives. Marjoram's antiseptic properties make it a good facial cleanser, and it has been used in cosmetic facial waters.

This familiar kitchen herb has a delicate and sweet flavor similar to oregano with a hint of balsam. You'll find it paired with poultry and beef, and complementing stews, sautés, potato dishes, and marinades. But marjoram's value goes beyond the kitchen. Contained within its gray-green, velvety leaves is a powerhouse of antimicrobial compounds.

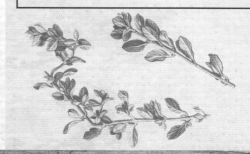

Broad-Spectrum Protection

Marjoram is a broad antioxidant and antimicrobial. Not only have studies shown that marjoram inhibits several viruses, including the herpes virus, it has also been confirmed that the herb is effective against fungi and bacteria. In one study, the microbicidal effects of a methanol extract of *Origanum majorana L.* (sweet marjoram) were tested on both fungi *(Fusarium solani, Candida albicans, Aspergillus niger, A. parasiticus, Rhizopus oryzae, Rhizoctonia otyzae-sativae and Altemaria brassicicola)* and bacteria *(Bacillus subtilis, B. megaterium, Escherichia coli, Proteus vulgaris, Pseudomonas aeruginosa and Staphylococcus aureus)*. It was found to be an effective protectant against all pathogens. The steam-distilled volatile oil also has strong inhibitory powers against common bacteria.

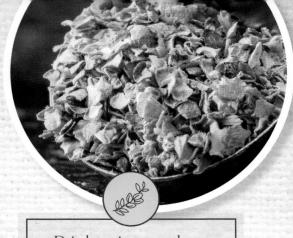

Dried marjoram makes a fine mild tea, though it is not as medicinally potent as the fresh plant.

Marjoram Essential Oil

Marjoram essential oil eases stiff joints and muscle spasms, including tics, excessive coughing, menstrual cramps, and headaches (especially migraines). It also slightly lowers high blood pressure. Testing has shown it to be one of the most effective fragrances in relaxing brain waves. As a result, it makes an excellent calming massage oil, delightful when combined with the softer lavender. Add a few drops to your bath to counter stress or insomnia. Since it has specific properties that fight the viruses and bacteria responsible for colds, flu, or laryngitis, add a few drops of essential oil to either a chest balm or bath, or put 2 or 3 drops in a bowl of hot water and inhale the steam. In healing salves and creams, it also soothes burns, bruises, and inflammation. The diluted essential oil can be rubbed into sore gums, in place of clove oil. Breathing the oil can help clear mucous from the lungs. A single drop in a glass of water can improve digestion.

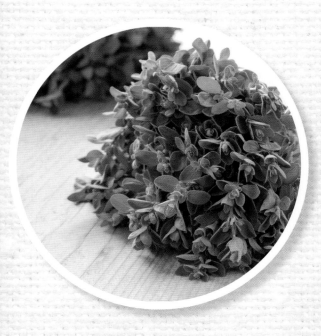

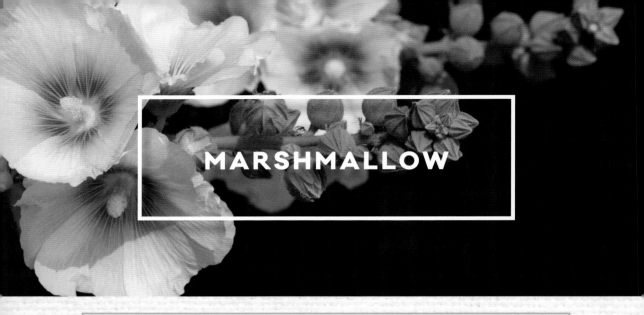

MARSHMALLOW

BOTANICAL NAME: *ALTHEA OFFICINALIS*

Yes, those popular campfire confections originated with these lovely plants. The Greeks used marshmallow to treat wounds, toothaches, coughing, and insect stings. The Romans valued marshmallow roots and leaves for their laxative properties. And during the Renaissance, marshmallow was used extensively to treat sore throats, stomach problems, and even venereal diseases. Marshmallow is a wonderful demulcent that soothes digestive tract inflammations and irritations; it helps heals stomach ulcers. It is also used in formulas to treat urinary and prostate infections and inflammations. It enhances immunity by stimulating white blood cells. Applied as a poultice, it helps to heal cuts and bruises. The roots are sometimes used in salves and poultices. In the kitchen, add uncooked young tops and tender leaves to spring salads, or fry roots with butter and onions.

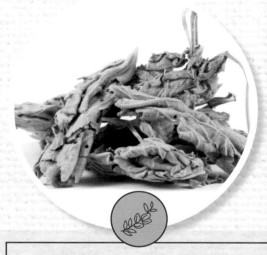

Dried marshmallow leaves, steeped as a tea, act as an expectorant and relieve lung dryness. The leaves are also a diuretic and soothe the urinary tract. Drink marshmallow tea to soothe the irritation of coughs and sore throats.

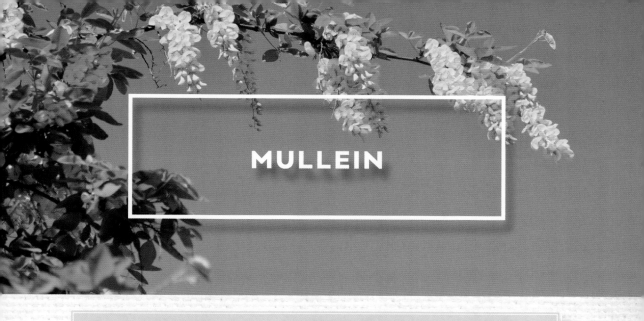

MULLEIN

BOTANICAL NAME: *VERBASCUM THAPSUS*

For centuries, mullein was considered an amulet against witches and evil spirits. The plant has many uses—both medicinal and household. For example, the dried stems were dipped in suet and burned as torches. For centuries, mullein's leaves have been used to heal lung conditions. Herbalists once even recommended that patients with lung diseases smoke dried, crumbled mullein leaves. Ayurvedic physicians prescribed mullein to treat coughs. And colonists considered mullein so valuable they brought it with them to America, where Indians eventually adopted it for treating coughs, bronchitis, and asthma.

Contemporary herbalists still recommend the internal use of mullein leaves to treat colds, sore throat, and coughs. The flowers and leaves can reduce inflammation in the urinary and digestive tract and treat colitis, intestinal bleeding, and diarrhea. The fresh flower infused alone or with garlic in olive oil makes an ear oil for pain and inflammation associated with an earache. In fact, herbalists repeatedly note that mullein oil effectively combats earaches and ear infections.

We now know that mullein has antiseptic and antiviral properties. A paste of mullein flowers can be applied to wounds and scrapes. In one study, compounds extracted from mullein were effective against the Herpes simplex virus type 1. Mullein extract also appears to inhibit a number of bacteria, including *Klebsiella pneumoniae*, *Staphylococcus aureus*, and *Staphylococcus epidermidis*.

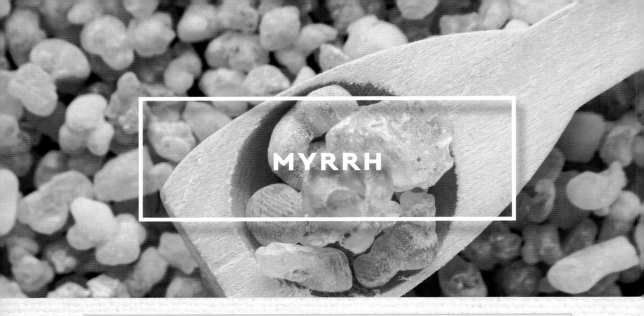

MYRRH

BOTANICAL NAME: *COMMIPHORA MYRRHA*

This small, scrubby, spiny tree from the Middle East and North East Africa is not very handsome, but it makes up for its looks with the precious gum it exudes. An important trade item for several thousand years, myrrh was a primary ingredient in ancient cosmetics and incenses. Believed to comfort sorrow, its name means "bitter tears." This may also refer to the bitter-tasting myrrh sap, which oozes in drops when the tree's bark is cut. Myrrh was added to wine by both the Greeks and Hebrews to heighten sensual awareness. The yellow to amber-colored oil is distilled from the gum and frequently added to toothpastes and gum preparations to help alleviate mouth ulcers, gum inflammation, and infection.

Myrrh is an expensive but effective treatment for chapped, cracked, or aged skin, eczema, bruises, infection, varicose veins, ringworm, and athlete's foot. Included in many ointments, it dries weepy wounds. It is a specific remedy for mouth and gum disease and is found in many oral preparations. It is very helpful applied on herpes sores and blisters: Add it to a lip balm, using about 25 drops per ounce. Lozenges or syrup containing myrrh treat coughs. As an additional bonus, it increases the activity of the immune system.

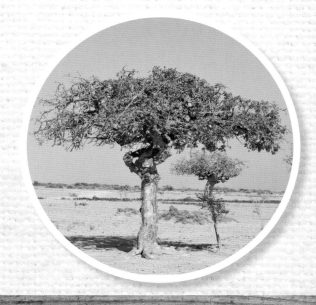

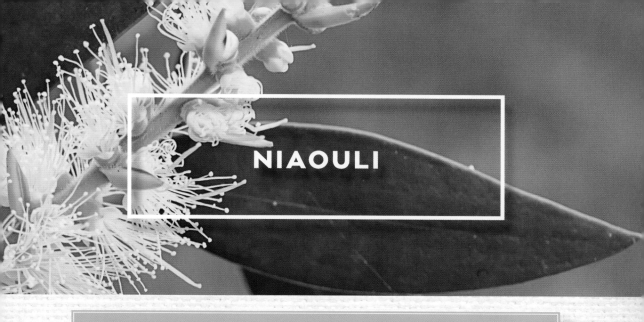

NIAOULI

BOTANICAL NAME: *MELALEUCA QUINQUENERVIA*

Niaouli is one of several names used for a tree found in Australia, New Guinea, and nearby islands. It has now been spread to many other parts of the world. Niaouli is also the most common name given to the essential oil from this tree. Human medicinal usage began with indigenous Australians, who used the bruised leaves to treat sickness. They also used parts of the tree to disinfect water.

The essential oil of niaouli is an incredibly powerful antibiotic, antifungal, and antiviral. It can be added to homemade cleaning blends where a strong disinfectant is needed. It is also an excellent oil to have on hand during cold and flu season—steam inhalation, diffusion, or use in the shower is a popular way to use the oil to help ward off viral bugs. On its own, the oil is a strong-smelling decongestant. That said, niaouli is not considered a completely pleasant-smelling essential oil. It has a peculiar medicinal aroma that can take getting used to.

Niaouli is related to tea tree and the two essential oils share a number of properties. Niaouli can often be substituted for tea tree when using it in topical applications. For many people, it is a gentler, less irritating oil. It is excellent for treating boils, cuts, and insect bites. It also effectively treats oily, dull, or acne-prone skin.

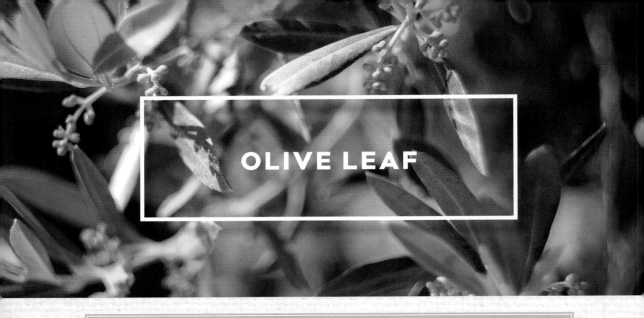

OLIVE LEAF

BOTANICAL NAME: *OLEA EUROPAEA*

The olive tree is native to the Mediterranean basin. Cultivation of olive trees goes back at least 7,000 years. Traditional healers used the leaf in poultice and decoction form to reduce fevers and fight infections. Even though olive leaf's use as a medicinal food and general tonic goes back to ancient Egypt, it has tended to be overlooked in traditional herbalism. In this century it has finally become fairly well known. Olive leaf teas, tinctures, extracts, and capsules can now be found online and at health food stores.

Olive leaf is broad in its effects: it combats bacteria, viruses, and fungi. Recent research reveals that compounds in olive leaf interfere with the proteins in virus particles, reducing their ability to infect us. It slows viral replication by preventing budding or assembly at the cell membrane. Olive leaf also seems to stimulate the immune system, and the activity of white blood cells in particular. A traditional remedy for sore throats is a strong olive tea gargle. Olive leaf extract has been shown to be effective against candida.

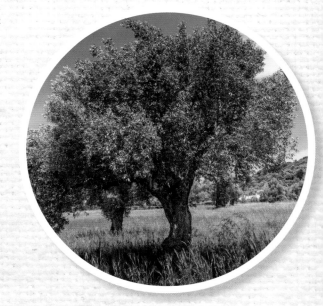

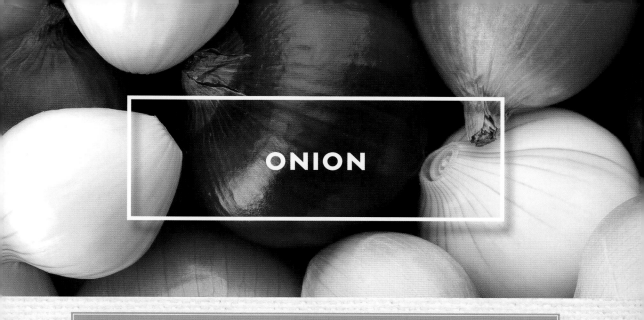

ONION

BOTANICAL NAME: *ALLIUM CEPA*

The onion is one of the oldest cultivated plants known. Traditional remedies employing onions abound in every culture where they are a food source. Although less research has been done on onions than on garlic, findings show the two have many of the same properties. Onions are excellent at killing bacteria and viruses. Their antimicrobial properties help fight infections.

A mixture of onion juice and honey is potent traditional cure for common colds, coughs, and sore throats. A simple cough syrup can be made by chopping several onions and combining them with sugar and storing them in a jar for half a day. The resulting strained liquid can be stored and doled out by the teaspoon as needed.

Food Is Medicine

Onions are a top-rate medicinal food. A Harvard Medical School study showed that "good" HDL cholesterol climbed significantly when participants ate about half of a medium-sized raw onion each day. Cooked onion did not affect HDL levels. Like garlic, onions also contain the smooth-muscle relaxant adenosine. This means that onions, too, may fight high blood pressure. They play a role in preventing blood clots as well, keeping blood platelets from sticking together and quickly dissolving clots that may have already formed. Researchers in India found that when raw or cooked onions were eaten along with fatty foods, the blood's clot-dissolving ability remained intact, which doesn't usually occur after fatty foods are eaten. It's a good idea, then, always to include onions when you eat that occasional high-fat meal. Be aware, though, that onions may cause heartburn to worsen in some people.

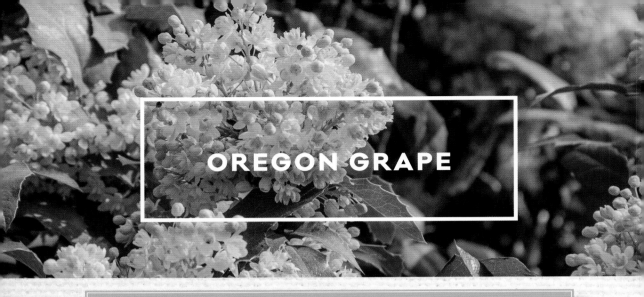

OREGON GRAPE

BOTANICAL NAME: *BERBERIS AQUIFOLIUM*

Oregon grape grows on the west coast of North America, from British Columbia to California. The plant was used by indigenous people in the region for digestive problems and skin conditions. A tea made from the root was used to ease arthritis and diarrhea.

Depending on need, the root, root-like stem, or berries may be used to make medicine. Oregon grape's prime constituent, the alkaloid berberine, is both an antibiotic and antifungal. It effectively kills giardia and candida organisms and several other intestinal parasites, which are responsible for intestinal upsets and vaginal yeast infections. Oregon grape root is useful to treat serious cases of diarrhea and digestive tract infection. It is also an exceptionally effective treatment for colds, flu, and numerous other infections. In the laboratory, it's been shown to kill or suppress the growth of several disease-causing microbes. The berberine compounds make it a good douche and skin cleanser for infections. The tincture is an effective treatment for eczema, acne, herpes, and psoriasis. Berberine will slow unhealthy skin's abnormal cell growth and reduce inflammation. Minor skin wounds can be treated with tincture. Eye conditions like conjunctivitis and sties can be treated topically by applying a diluted tea to the area.

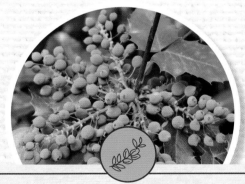

High in vitamin C, the berries may be eaten raw or cooked in jam. Berries are also used to flavor jelly, wine, and soups. They have been used in folk medicine and seem to have some of the same medicinal properties as the root, but they are probably not as potent.

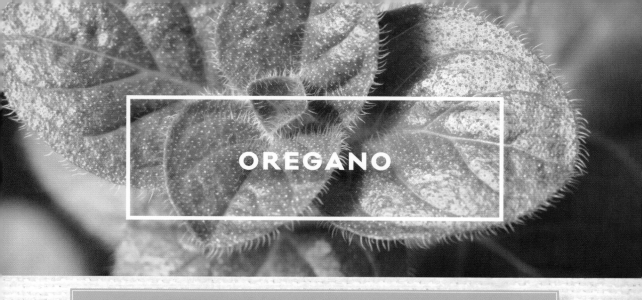

OREGANO

BOTANICAL NAME: *ORIGANUM VULGARE*

The culinary herb we associate with Italian cuisine and pizza seasoning has a medicinal side that may surprise you. Oregano has been cultivated for thousands of years. It originates in the Mediterranean region. The Greeks are credited with first using oregano, and the name itself comes from Greek words meaning "mountain joy." It was used as both a food herb and a general tonic. The raw leaves were chewed to ease rheumatism, toothache, indigestion, and lingering coughs. It became known across ancient cultures for its tonic, antispasmodic, stomachic, and cough-suppressing virtues.

Today, the essential oil is especially prized for its antibiotic properties. In one notable experiment, the diluted oil was added to a cultivated mixture of sewer water and beef broth. Researchers were astonished to find that it completely sterilized the water. Multiple studies have confirmed that the essential oil of oregano is remarkably strong—outperforming pharmaceutical antibiotics in a number of cases. It destroys or inhibits the growth of a broad spectrum of pathogens, including *E. coli, Staphylococcus aureus, Listeria innocua, Saccharomyces cerevisiae, Aspergillus niger, Bacillus cereus, Bacillus subtilis, Candida albicans,* and *Eimeria tenella,* just to name a few.

Two compounds in oregano essential oil stand out as exceptional: carvacrol and para-cymene. These antibiotic substances are effective against all four classes of pathogens. And not only does oregano have these broad-spectrum effects against all four groups, it is also known to boost immune function.

Oregano is much more than a flavorful kitchen herb. It packs impressive broad-spectrum effects that include antibacterial, antifungal, antiviral, antiparasitic, antioxidant, and anti-inflammatory properties.

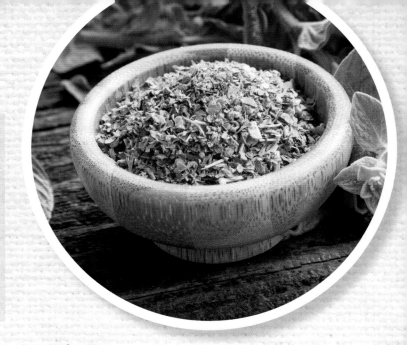

Oregano Tea

Oregano is related to marjoram, and so it isn't surprising that oregano tea is used for some of the same purposes as marjoram tea. A simple tea, using either the fresh or dried herb, is drunk for coughs, nausea, digestive problems, irritable bowel syndrome, and just about every respiratory ailment. One recipe for warding off colds and the flu uses a tablespoon of chopped ginger, boiled in two cups of water for several minutes. 10 fresh oregano leaves are then added to the liquid. Once the mixture has cooled slightly, a tablespoon of honey is stirred in. The mixture is then strained and drunk.

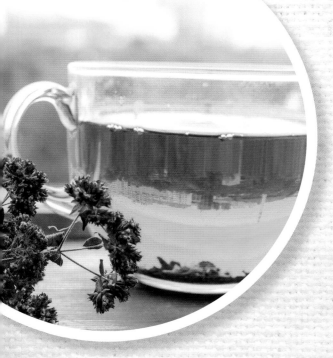

Oregano Essential Oil

• **Foot and nail fungus:** Mix 3 drops oregano oil, 2 drops thyme oil, and 10 drops carrier oil (like coconut) and apply the mixture twice daily.

• **Thrush:** Mix 2 drops oregano oil with 15 drops carrier oil. Swab mixture inside mouth.

• **Laundry:** Add 3 drops oregano oil per single load to laundry detergent to help kill bacteria and eliminate bacterial smells.

• **Acne:** Mix 2 drops oregano oil with 1 teaspoon aloe vera gel and apply to problem area with a cotton swab.

• **Sinus infections and colds:** Add a few drops to your shower (someplace where the oil won't immediately wash away) and allow the oil to mingle with the steam.

• **Warts:** Dilute 1 drop oregano oil in a small amount of carrier oil and apply directly on wart. Cover with bandage. Repeat and replace bandage daily until wart disappears.

• **Mouthwash:** Add a few drops to a glass of water and gargle with the liquid to kill bacteria and sweeten breath.

• **Bathtub mold:** Mix 10 drops oregano oil with 14 ounces water in a spray bottle and spray area affected by the mold.

• **Kitchen disinfectant:** Add several drops to your kitchen cleaner to bolster its antimicrobial power.

Oregano Is for the Birds

In 2012, a study noted that commercial chicken farmers are increasingly turning to cinnamon and oregano oil in lieu of problematic pharmaceutical antibiotics. The move is proving to be a viable alternative—the natural antibiotic properties of these essential oils are keeping the chickens healthy and disease-free. And it's not just chickens: pig, sheep, and cattle farmers have noted the success and are experimenting with substituting oregano and other essential oils into their feed regimen.

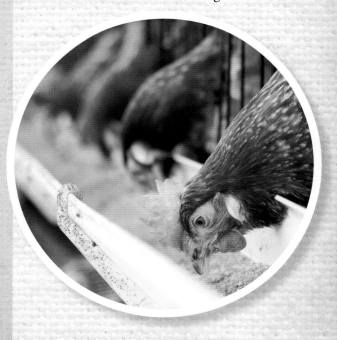

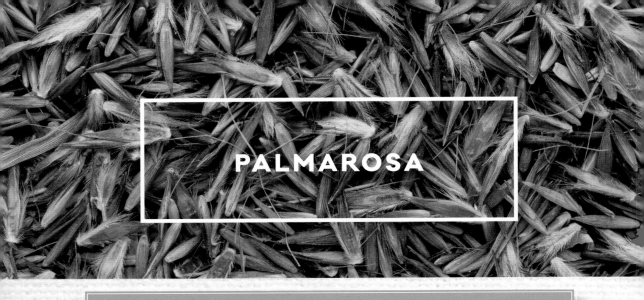

PALMAROSA

BOTANICAL NAME: *CYMBOPOGON MARTINII*

Native to India, palmarosa is a species of grass that is often cultivated specifically for its aromatic, sweet, rose-scented oil. In fact, it was given the name "palmarosa"—which means "palm rose"—thanks to its lovely scent. Traditionally, the oil was used to keep insects away from stores of grains and beans, and for treating infections and aches and pains. The leaves were crushed and made into poultices, and the grass and roots were steeped into tea and taken for bronchitis, fevers, and jaundice. Palmarosa is popular in the perfume and cosmetic industry, and its oil is especially prized for its skin-loving properties.

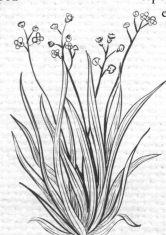

The oil is excellent for skin care, increasing hydration in the skin and promoting cell growth. Palmarosa's aromatic scent makes it a perfect choice for soaps, lotions, and cosmetics. But palmarosa has much more to offer than a sweet scent and a skin ally.

The essential oil usually contains around 70 percent geraniol, whose antibiotic activity is especially strong against bacteria, viruses, and fungi. It can be used topically to combat just about any type of skin infection, and is useful for treating conditions like eczema and psoriasis. The oil helps to increase stomach acid, which aids healthy digestion. It can be diluted and taken internally for digestive and urinary tract disorders.

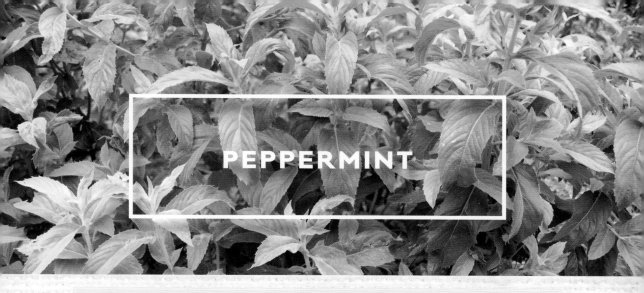

PEPPERMINT

BOTANICAL NAME: *MENTHA PIPERITA*

One of the most widely used of all aromatics, peppermint makes a grand and obvious appearance in all sorts of products, including beverages, ice cream, liqueurs, medicines, dental preparations, cleaners, desserts, and gums. After the *British Medical Journal* noted in 1879 that smelling menthol (the main component in peppermint) relieves headaches and nerve pain, menthol cones that evaporate into the air became all the rage. Taking center stage in several controversies, herbalists have long argued for or against the assertion by the ancient Greek physician Galen that peppermint is an aphrodisiac. But everyone, including modern scientists, agrees that it is a strong mental and physical stimulant that can help one concentrate and stay awake and alert.

Therapeutically, peppermint is a truly broad-spectrum workhorse. It is an anti-inflammatory and relieves muscle spasms and cramping. Peppermint is an excellent intestinal tonic, decreasing gas and indigestion, relieving flatulence, and easing stomach cramps. It actually relaxes the digestive muscles so they operate more efficiently. A massage over the abdomen with an oil containing peppermint can greatly aid intestinal spasms, indigestion, nausea, and irritable bowel syndrome. Peppermint relieves the itching of ringworm, herpes simplex, scabies, and poison oak. Simply smelling the essential oil can clear sinus and lung congestion while killing some viral infections and many bacteria.

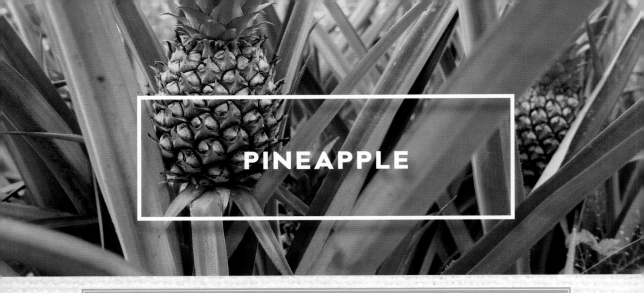

PINEAPPLE

BOTANICAL NAME: *ANANAS COMOSUS*

The fruit of a low-growing, tropical plant native to Central and South America, pineapple is now cultivated in tropical regions throughout the world. While it is commonly considered simply a tasty ingredient in desserts and fruit dishes, pineapple contains an array of health-promoting compounds that can fight illness and boost immunity.

The key compound in pineapple is bromelain, an enzyme that has antiviral and antibacterial properties and appears to have a general tonic effect on multiple systems in the body. Anecdotally, its antibacterial effects are reported most effective against mouth- and throat-related ailments. It helps to suppress coughs, loosen mucus in the throat, and ease illness-related respiratory inflammation. It also soothes the symptoms of allergies and asthma.

Tastiest Cough Syrup Ever?

One classic natural cough suppressant recipe consists of one cup of pineapple juice, the juice of one lemon, a large piece of finely minced ginger, a tablespoon of honey, and a half teaspoon of ground cayenne pepper. The ingredients are combined and the concoction sipped as needed.

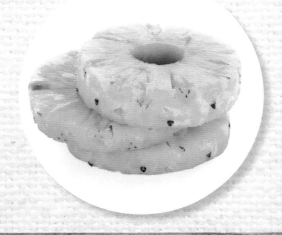

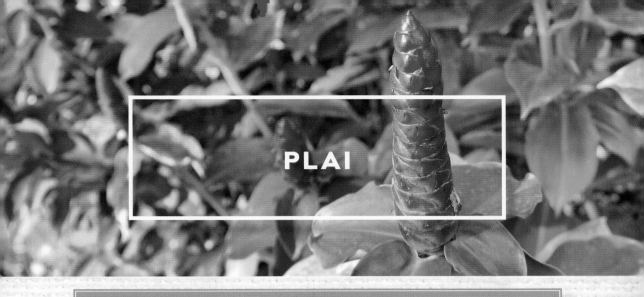

PLAI

BOTANICAL NAME: *ZINGIBER CASSUMUNAR*

Native to Thailand, plai is a species of plant in the same family as ginger. Although not well known in the United States, the essential oil of plai has long been used by Thai massage therapists due to its ability to relieve discomfort and inflammation. Unlike ginger, plai has a pleasant cooling effect that makes it especially soothing for aches and pains.

The oil has a very high concentration of a substance called Terpinen-4-ol, which is the same ingredient that gives tea tree oil its antimicrobial properties—making plai another all-purpose pathogen fighter.

Plai's anti-inflammatory properties make it especially effective for treating aches and pains associated with muscle pulls and strains. It can be used to prevent infection and treat skin conditions such as acne. When used in a diffuser, plai has been shown to be helpful for asthma, bronchitis, and colds and flu. Its antispasmodic properties help to ease menstrual pain and irritable bowel syndrome.

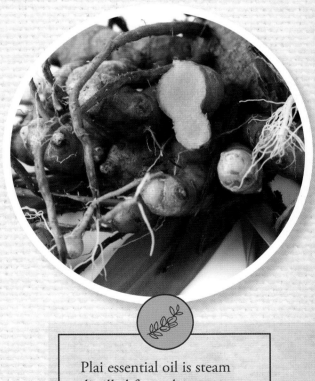

Plai essential oil is steam distilled from the roots.

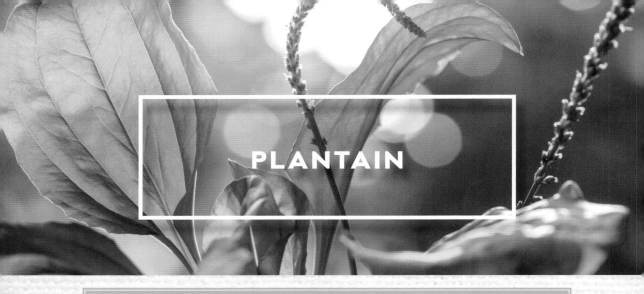

PLANTAIN

BOTANICAL NAME: *PLANTAGO MAJOR*

Homeowners who strive for the perfect lawn may consider this ubiquitous plant a nuisance, but plantain is a powerful healer that is worth our respect. It has been used for centuries to treat a variety of ailments. The ancient Saxons, in fact, regarded plantain as one of the most essential herbs in cultivation. If a bee stings you, apply crushed, fresh plantain leaves to the welt, which will soon disappear. And if you stumble into a patch of poison ivy, you needn't scratch and suffer. Apply a poultice of plantain leaves to relieve your discomfort. Some people, moreover, have been known to chew plantain root to stop the pain of a toothache.

A mild diuretic, the herb is useful for treating urinary problems. Lung disorders, such as asthma and bronchitis, also respond to plantain. Research from India shows that it reduces the symptoms of colds and coughs and relieves the pain and wheezing associated with bronchial problems.

Plantain is a forgotten kitchen herb. Although the leaves are fairly fibrous, small amounts can be added fresh to salads. The tender young leaves can be steamed like spinach. The seeds are edible. Add small amounts to other grains to increase protein. The species *P. psyllium* is a popular laxative; it is used, as is *P. ovata*, in products such as Metamucil. As with other foods that provide bulk, it has been shown to reduce cholesterol levels.

Applied externally, the plant stimulates and cleanses the skin and encourages wounds to heal faster. Plantain has also been used to dye wool a dull gold or camel color.

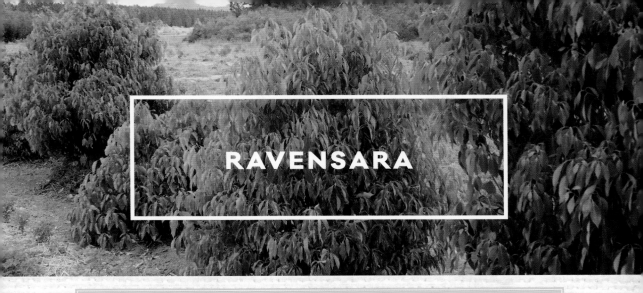

RAVENSARA

BOTANICAL NAME: *RAVENSARA AROMATICA*

Undeservedly obscure, ravensara's distilled leaves yield an essential oil that is a standout antiviral. Though not much to look at, the tree thrives in the humid rain forests of Madagascar, where people traditionally burned the leaves to help ward off disease.

Aromatherapists recommend having "the oil that heals" around during the winter cold and flu season. Add a few drops to a hot bath or shower, inhale it via diffuser, or simply carry a vial around with you and take a whiff when needed. Ravensara stimulates the immune system and bronchi, neutralizes microbes, and soothes lungs and sinuses. It enhances immunity-boosting blends and works well with oils like chamomile, cypress, eucalyptus, lavender, lemon, marjoram, niaouli, rosemary, and thyme. It also helps relieve the irritation of chicken pox and shingles.

Ravensara or Ravintsara?

It's not just a variant spelling for the same oil—there is an essential oil named ravintsara, and it is a distinctly different oil. Ravintsara is derived from a specific kind of *Cinnamomum camphora* tree. While its therapeutic uses overlap with those of ravensara (via inhalation, it's a great antiviral that can alleviate cold, flu, and respiratory conditions), its chemical profile is different. Correct identifcation of the two essential oils in the marketplace has been spotty over the past several decades. When you purchase ravensara, make sure that your source identifies the oil as *ravensara aromatica*, and that the retailer is clearly distinguishing between the two oils.

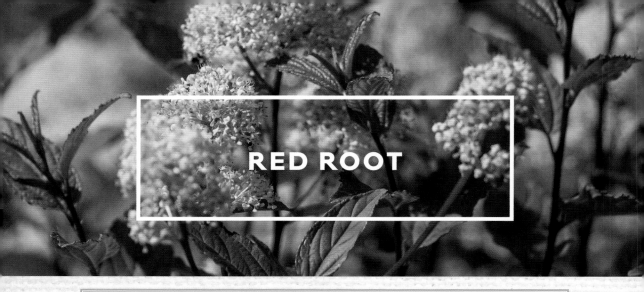

RED ROOT

BOTANICAL NAME: *CEANOTHUS AMERICANUS*

Sometimes called New Jersey tea, red root is a hardy, deep-rooted plant native to eastern North America. Native Americans used the root for a wide variety of ailments, including colds and coughs, and to treat digestive problems and lung conditions. American Eclectic physicians adopted the use of red root in the mid-19th century. It is still used in the folk medicine of Appalachia to treat sore throats.

While red root is most commonly used to address deficiencies in the lymphatic system (to reduce lymphatic swelling and strengthen lymph tissue, for example), it is also used for its antibacterial and antiviral properties. Red root contains triterpenes and flavonoids, which help make the body environment less hospitable to invaders. Although red root is considered an antiviral, it does not specifically kill viruses. Instead it bolsters the lymphatic system by speeding movement of fluids through the lymph and also decreases swelling of the liver and spleen. It has been used to combat mumps, mononucleosis, and rocky mountain fever. Its constituents ceanothic acid and ceanothetric acid have specifically been shown to inhibit the growth of the pathogens *Actinomyces viscosus, P. gingivalis,* and *Streptococcus mutans* in laboratory experiments. (A tincture must be used, rather than a tea, to take advantage of the anti-streptococcal activity, however.) In tea form, red root is astringent. The anti-inflammatory and antimicrobial constituents in the tea help soothe and disinfect sore throats. Red root tea effectively accelerates the healing process after bouts of pharyngitis, tonsillitis, and nasal catarrh.

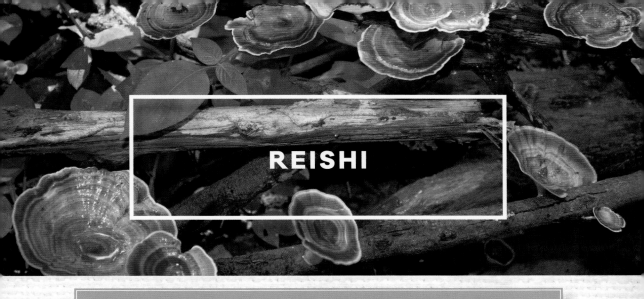

REISHI

BOTANICAL NAME: *GANODERMA LUCIDUM*

The reishi mushroom grows wild in the temperate forests of Asia and can be found in the northeastern United States growing on hemlock trees. Its cap can grow up to a foot wide and an inch or two thick. Reishi might lead all medicinal mushrooms in one category: number of nicknames. A fixture of eastern medicine for at least four thousand years, it is often called the "queen of mushrooms" due to what some consider to be powerful effects on the health of both mind and body. Traditional Chinese medical literature called it the "spirit plant" and the "tree of life mushroom." The Japanese have variously termed it "mushroom of immortality," "good fortune mushroom," and "ten-thousand-year mushroom."

In traditional Chinese medicine, reishi has been used for a vast array of ailments and could be considered a general panacea. It was prescribed for liver problems, asthma, bronchitis, nephritis of the kidneys, nerve pain, ulcers, and insomnia.

Unlike many other medicinal mushrooms, reishi is not typically included on the lunch or dinner menu. It has a hard, woody texture and a bitter taste, and thus is usually taken as a powder, extract or supplement. Those who can handle its bitter taste can certainly brew reishi tea or consume it with coffee.

All-purpose Tonic

Like many other medicinal mushrooms, reishi varieties are thought to be effective because they are packed with antioxidants. The compounds within the reishi have been linked in some studies to (among others) improved function in the immune system, lower cholesterol, reduced inflammation, regulated blood pressure, increased strength and stamina, and even cancer fighting and prevention.

There are many who swear by reishi for a wellness benefit not common to many other medicinal mushrooms—help with fatigue. While there is no hard science to support this claim, reishi has been linked to better energy and stamina.

One side effect must be noted: reishi has been known to cause toxicity in some immune cells, and there have been documented cases of liver toxicity. Other side effects can include mouth, throat and nasal passage dryness, itching, upset stomach, and nosebleeds.

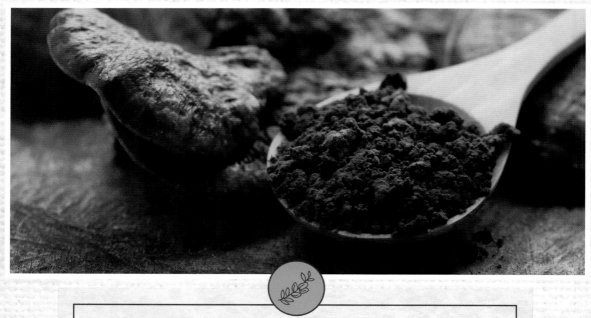

Dried reishi is quite hard, due to the chitin that makes up the cell walls. A long hot-water extraction is necessary to break the chitin down and unlock the medicinal molecules. Reishi should be broken into smaller pieces or ground into a powder before adding it to water. The resulting tea is too bitter for some people. Luckily, reishi supplements in capsule form are readily available.

A Long List of Benefits

Inflammation and immune system: Most studies linking the reishi mushroom to better immune system function have been done in test tube situations or with compromised cells of those with illnesses. However, some claim reishi mushrooms can bolster wellness in healthy people, too. It has been tested on athletes in stressful situations (elevated heart rate, muscle fatigue, and other sport-induced states). Other studies have looked into whether reishi can even help those suffering bad allergy symptoms "breathe easier" due to substances called triterpenes in the mushrooms. Research is young. What has been consistent is the impact of reishi mushrooms on white blood cells and as an anti-inflammatory agent.

Cancer prevention/treatment: Complex sugars called beta-glucans found in reishi might possess the ability to stop cancer cells from growing or spreading. There are no truly convincing studies involving human cells to pronounce reishi a cancer-fighter just yet. One study did show that an unusually high percentage of breast cancer survivors took reishi as a supplement. And there is ongoing research into reishi and its potential impact against prostate cancer due to its effects on testosterone. Some of the most promising cancer tests around reishi have studied whether it might work well in conjunction with traditional treatments.

Heart disease: Studies suggest that taking reishi mushrooms might correlate with an increase in HDL "good" cholesterol and a reduction in triglycerides. Other studies have disputed these results. There is ongoing research into the impact of reishi on blood pressure, another contributing factor to good heart health, due to triterpenes found in reishi mushrooms.

Fatigue, depression, stamina issues: This is a broad area, and perhaps the one where reishi stands out among other medicinal mushrooms. Many believe that the reishi mushroom can be effective in improving mental health, energy, and stamina. One of the oft-cited studies in this regard tested 132 people suffering from aches, pains, irritability, and dizziness. Researchers noted that after eight weeks of taking reishi supplements, their patients experienced improved well-being and reduced fatigue.

Other studies have associated reishi with an ability to sleep more soundly, which can improve energy, reduce fatigue, and contribute to better mental health. One four-week study of 48 breast cancer survivors showed that taking reishi powder daily might have reduced their fatigue and decreased feelings of anxiety and depression. Many reported an improved quality of life.

The medical community still points out that there is little in the way of scientific evidence to support reishi as a proven treatment for fatigue, sleep disorders, anxiety, depression, or even weight loss (another area where reishi is being studied). Still, many swear by a daily dose of reishi supplement for improved overall mental, physical, and even spiritual health. Thousands of years of eastern medicine are on their side.

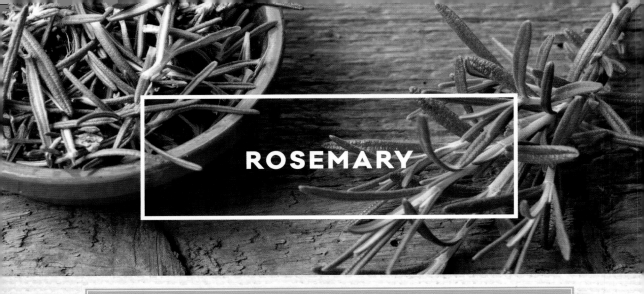

ROSEMARY

This Mediterranean native with tiny, pale blue flowers that bloom in late winter loves growing by the ocean—its latin name rosmarinus means "dew of the sea." It is cultivated worldwide, although France, Spain, and Tunisia are the main producers of the essential oil. Rosemary has been used as a medicinal herb throughout recorded history. It was a common garden herb during the Roman Empire. The ancient Greeks, Egyptians, and Hebrews cultivated it as well.

Before refrigeration, cooks wrapped meat in rosemary leaves to preserve it. Though it can have an overpoweringly pungent taste—reminiscent of both mint and ginger—its aroma has come to be associated with Mediterranean cuisines. It complements poultry, fish, lamb, beef, veal, pork, game, cheese, and eggs, as well as many vegetables, including potatoes, tomatoes, spinach, and mushrooms. While efforts have been made to tap rosemary's strong antibacterial properties for commercial food preservation, the herb's strong piney aroma has thus far prevented widespread usage.

As an antibacterial, rosemary is good for more than food preservation. A gargle of diluted rosemary oil and water relieves sore throats, gum problems, and canker sores. Another way to relieve lung congestion and sore throat is to inhale the essential oil directly or via diffusion, or add it to a vapor balm that is rubbed on the chest and throat. Either the whole-plant extract or the diluted essential oil can be applied to acne to kill the bacteria and reduce the associated inflammation. Rosemary is a good general tonic for the skin as well; the oil and herb are added to cosmetics to improve skin tone. It encourages dry, mature skin to produce more of its own natural oils. The herb makes a fragrant, refreshing bath additive and hair rinse. It stimulates the scalp and helps control dandruff.

Rosemary promotes digestion and stimulates the activity of the liver and gallbladder to aid both in digestion of fats and the detoxification of the body. It also inhibits the formation of kidney stones. The herb has been prescribed topically to treat muscle spasms. Rosemary oil helps reduce the pain of rheumatism when used as a liniment. It can be applied to eczema and wounds. It strengthens blood vessels and improves circulation, so it is useful to treat varicose veins and other problems related to poor circulation. For this reason, it can also relieve some headaches. A foot bath containing rosemary is good for swollen ankles and feet that tend to be numb or cold often—both signs of poor circulation.

In the kitchen, rosemary essential oil is a good disinfectant boost to cleaning agents. It has robust antibacterial properties and tests have shown that the oil inhibits the growth of *E. coli*, *Listeria monocytogenes,* and *Staphylococcus aureus.* In addition, the oil has a number of antifungal mechanisms which inhibit a number of fungi.

Fresh Rosemary Tea

Fresh rosemary—whether from your garden or the grocery store—packs a potent array of antioxidants. Steeping a twig of fresh rosemary in a pot of simmering water for ten minutes unleashes the plant's benefits and provides a delicious herbal tea. Rosemary is an astringent, expectorant, and diaphoretic (induces sweating). Because of this, it is an especially useful tea to drink when you're suffering through a cold. Drink it three times a day until your cold is gone. Ginger, lemon, and manuka honey (added after the tea has cooled) are good additions to this concoction.

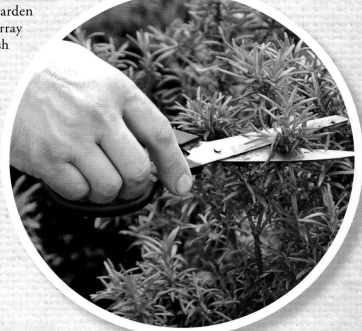

Easy to grow, rosemary is an attractive, spreading evergreen. Its needle-shaped leaves may be pruned to form a low hedge.

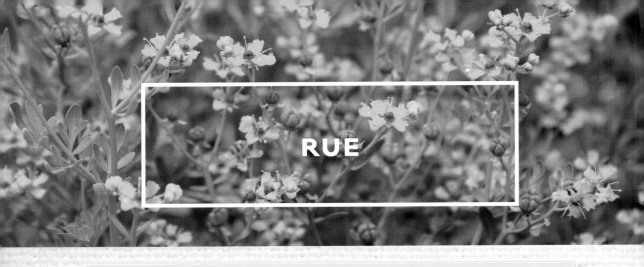

RUE

BOTANICAL NAME: *RUTA GRAVEOLENS*

The Greeks believed that rue cured nervous indigestion, improved eyesight, was an antidote to poison, and treated insect bites. Today, rue is more popular as a medicine in several countries other than the United States. The exception is the Latino community in the United States which uses *ruta* to relieve menstrual cramps and to regulate menstruation. Throughout Latin America, people use rue tea to treat colds and rue compresses applied to the chest to treat congestion. Rue is also used topically as a liniment to relieve the pain of rheumatoid arthritis and sore muscles.

In traditional Chinese medicine, rue is used to decrease the inflammation of sprains, strains, and bites. Rue contains rutin, which strengthens fragile blood vessels, so the herb helps diminish varicose veins and reduces bruising when used internally or topically. Rue eardrops decrease the pain and inflammation of an earache. Taken internally, rue relaxes muscles and nervous indigestion and improves circulation in the digestive tract. People in the Middle East use it to kill intestinal parasites, and in India, they say it improves mental clarity,

which is indeed possible because of its action on circulation.

Although it is bitter, minute amounts are used to flavor some baked goods. The Italians use rue as a bitter digestive, eating small amounts with other bitter greens and using it in a liqueur, *grappa con ruta*.

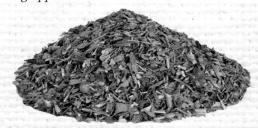

Dried rue leaves are used to repel pests like fleas, flies, roaches, and mosquitoes. While people do use the dried leaves for tea, it is best to only use in amounts recommended by a professional healthcare provider. The amounts should always be very small, and caution should be exercised due to the herb's toxicity.

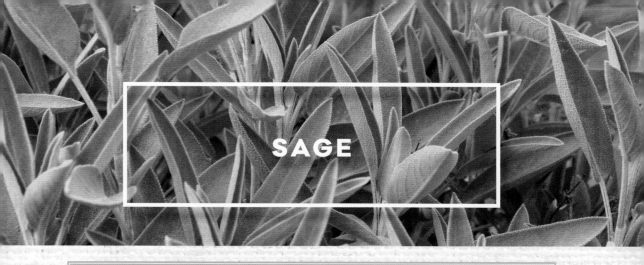

SAGE

BOTANICAL NAME: *SALVIA OFFICINALIS*

Sage is native to the Mediterranean and has been known for its medicinal properties since ancient times. Its name is derived from the Latin *salvere*, which means "to feel healthy" or "heal." This herb is one of the oldest-known plants used not only in medicine, but also in food. The Arabs associated sage with immortality, and the Greeks considered it an herb that promotes wisdom. Appropriately enough, a constituent in sage was recently discovered to inhibit an enzyme that produces memory loss and plays a role in Alzheimer's disease. However, it's unlikely that use of the herb alone will benefit these conditions.

Sage's essential oils have antiseptic properties, and the tannins are astringent. It has been used for centuries as a gargle for sore throat and inflamed gums. The herb is useful in treating cuts, and bruises. Sweating is decreased about two hours after ingesting sage; in fact, it is used in some deodorants, perfumes, cosmetics, and a German antiperspirant. It is also useful to prevent hot flashes, and it has some estrogenic properties. It decreases mother's milk so is useful while weaning children. It decreases saliva flow in the mouth and has successfully been used by people who have overactive salivary glands. It is a strong antioxidant and may prove useful against cell degeneration in the body. As a hair conditioner, a sage infusion reduces overactive glands in the scalp, which are sometimes responsible for causing dandruff. It also gives gloss to dark hair.

A Powerful Healer— in Moderation

Sage is excellent at preventing infections, both internal and external. Its antioxidant and anti-inflammatory properties make it a valuable ingredient for skin care, as it provides an anti-aging effect and helps fade scars. Sage oil provides relief from coughing and congestion, and it promotes the production of bile, which helps the digestive system to run smoothly. However, in large amounts, thujone, a constituent of sage, may cause a variety of symptoms, culminating in convulsions. For this reason, care must be taken when working with the essential oil of sage, which can have high concentrations of thujone. It is safe in the small amounts found in sage leaves.

Sage Tea

Sage tea has been a go-to remedy for sore throats, coughs, and respiratory ailments for millennia. The Greek physician Dioscorides (circa AD 40–90) noted its efficacy in his *De Materia Medica*. The tea's antimicrobial effects make it helpful for oral health. It kills common oral pathogens like *Streptococcus mutans* and candida. Sage tea also eases digestive problems, including flatulence, gastritis, diarrhea, bloating, and heartburn. The tea may be made from either fresh or dried sage.

Simple Sage Cough Syrup

This simple recipe is good to have around during cold and flu season. Combine 4 tablespoons chopped fresh sage, ¼ cup water, and the juice of 1 lemon in a saucepan and simmer on low heat for 10 minutes. Remove from heat, add 1 cup raw honey, and let steep for another 10 minutes. Strain and store the syrup in a clean glass jar. Use as needed for sore throats, colds, and coughs.

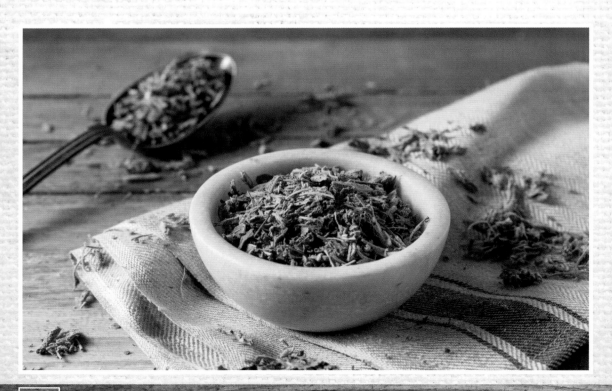

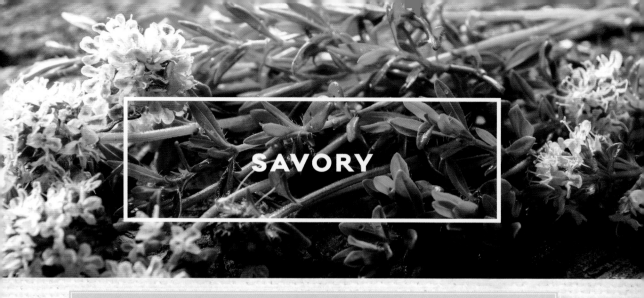

SAVORY

Summer savory is probably native to the Black Sea and eastern Mediterranean region. The Romans believed savory was sacred to satyrs. They planted it near beehives to increase honey production. They used savory to flavor vinegars and introduced the herb to England, where the Saxons adopted and named it for its spicy taste. Winter savory was said to curb sexual appetite; summer savory, to increase it. Guess which variety was most popular?

Summer savory has antiseptic and astringent properties, so it has been used to treat colic, asthma, and mild sore throats. Like many culinary herbs, it aids digestion, stimulates appetite, and relieves a minor upset stomach and eliminates gas—probably one reason it is so popular to flavor bean dishes. It also kills several types of intestinal worms. The herb is considered a good remedy for diarrhea. The essential oil contains a number of antibiotic substances, especially carvacrol, which boast extremely powerful, broad-spectrum action against all four classes of pathogens.

Summer's Cousin Winter

Winter savory (*Satureja montana*) may not be as popular as summer savory, but it is just as effective as a broad-spectrum antibiotic. The essential oil is extremely caustic—it should always be diluted before use. It may be used for infectious pathologies of the intestinal, respiratory, and urinary tract.

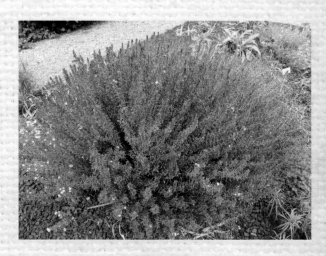

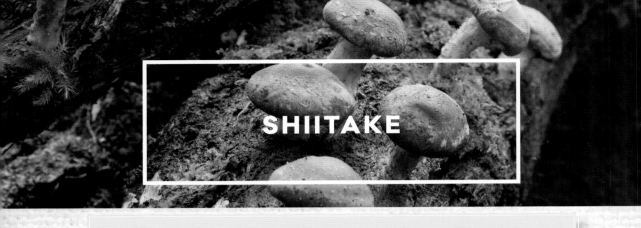

SHIITAKE

BOTANICAL NAME: *LENTINULA EDODES*

The shiitake may be the second-most consumed mushroom, after the button mushroom. Shiitake mushrooms have long been a staple of Chinese cuisine. They are eaten as medicinal food to increase stamina and general health, alleviate diabetes and high blood cholesterol, and boost immunity. In both China and Japan, shiitake mushrooms have been used for hundreds of years to fight cancer.

Juice extracted from shiitake mushrooms is an all-purpose pathogen fighter. In one study, it had a pronounced effect against *S. aureus, E. coli,* and *E. faecalis*, while leaving good intestinal bacteria alone. As an antiviral, it is effective against the common flu, avian flu virus (H5N1), and West Nile virus. Fermented shiitake has been used against *salmonella typhimurium*.

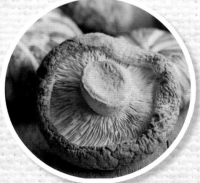

Research has found that lentinan, a chemical in shiitake mushrooms, slows the growth of cancerous tumors in animals. It activates the natural killer cells of the immune system and reduces prostaglandins responsible for inflammation. Lentinan is now used to enhance the human immune system and help people fight off cancer and infections. In Japan, it is used specifically in some breast cancer therapies. Lentinan has attracted attention in other areas as well. In one study, lentinan was tested against 29 bacteria and 10 fungi and found very effective against them.

Shiitake mushrooms also contain cortinelin, a strong antibacterial agent which kills a wide range of disease-causing germs. A sulfide compound extracted from shiitake mushrooms has also been found to have antibiotic properties. Shiitakes have been used to treat depressed immune-system disorders, including AIDS.

> It's easy to tap the health benefits of dried shiitakes. Simply pour boiling water over the minced caps, steep for 20 minutes and strain to make a quick tea. Steep them in warm water for a few hours and wash off any remaining dirt before cooking them.

Souped-Up Immunity

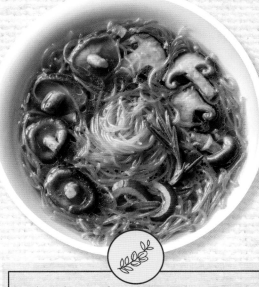

When the flu is making the rounds, add this simple homemade soup to your wellness regimen. It's packed with flavor and will give your immune system a helpful boost.

–1 medium white onion, chopped

–4 garlic cloves, chopped

–1 thumb-sized piece of fresh ginger, peeled and grated

–1 cup dried shiitake mushrooms

–Juice of 1 lemon

–1 tablespoon raw apple cider vinegar

–Salt, pepper, and red chili flakes to taste

–5 cups water

Soak and wash mushrooms first. Squeeze, pat dry, and slice them into strips, discarding the tough stem ends. In a soup pot, add all ingredients. Heat to a simmer, cover pot, and cook for two hours. Make the soup more substantial by adding ramen, udon, rice noodles, or egg noodles

Shiitake mushrooms are considered a superfood—a nutritious food source packed with protein and full of vitamins B1, B2, B12, niacin, and pantothenic acid. They can be eaten fresh or dried and reconstituted. They are full-flavored and slightly smoky-tasting, making great additions to soups, stews, and noodle dishes. Chinese physicians recommend eating 2 to 4 ounces of shiitake mushrooms two to three times a week to prevent cancer.

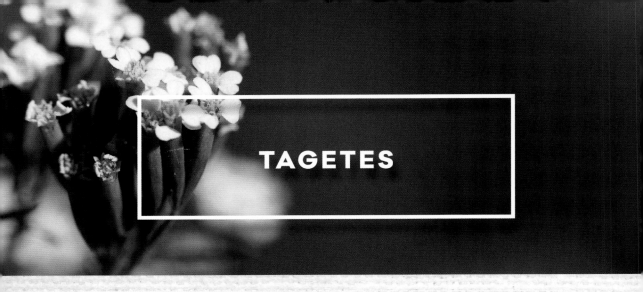

TAGETES

BOTANICAL NAME: *TAGETES MINUTA*

Also known as marigold, tagetes is a plant in the sunflower family native to North and South America; but many species—including *Tagetes minuta*, from which the essential oil is usually derived—have been naturalized around the world. The flowering plant grows well in just about any soil, and this attribute is what inspired its moniker: tagetes is derived from the name of the ancient Etruscan prophet Tages, who was said to have spontaneously sprung out of a plot of plowed ground. Tagetes is used as an herb and flavoring in many South American countries. Its flavor is described as a mix between basil, tarragon, mint, and citrus. The essential oil, which is steam distilled from the leaves, stalks, and flowers of the plant, has a sweet, fruity, slightly citrusy scent, and has traditionally been used to treat a myriad of ailments, including colds, whooping cough, colic, and mumps. This oil is often confused with calendula, but don't be fooled: tagetes is a gem in its own right.

Tagetes oil can be used to treat cuts and wounds and prevent infection, and is useful for treating and preventing fungal infections like athlete's foot. Its antibacterial and antifungal properties also make it a great disinfectant for your home, where it can be used to wipe down kitchen and bathroom countertops and floors. With its anti-inflammatory properties, tagetes is a great choice for easing aches and pains in joints and muscles, whether caused by arthritis, rheumatism, or injuries.

The oil has sedative effects which can calm coughs and spasms, and also help to relieve anxiety and stress. Tagetes has been used for centuries as a way to ease respiratory ailments, including colds, flu, and bronchitis. Add a few drops of tagetes oil to water and spray around your home to repel insects, including mosquitoes, fleas, and bedbugs.

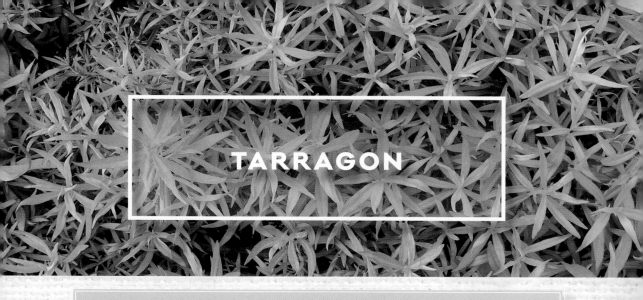

TARRAGON

BOTANICAL NAME: *ARTEMISIA DRACUNCULUS*

Written records of tarragon's use date back to at least 500 BC. Tarragon stimulates appetite, relieves gas and colic, and makes a good local anesthetic for toothaches (a fact first noted by the ancient Greeks). Tarragon has antifungal and antioxidant properties and has been used to preserve foods. It's also found in perfumes, soaps, cosmetics, condiments, and liqueurs. One of the French *fines herbes*, tarragon has a strong flavor that may overpower foods, so use it sparingly in salads and sauces, including remoulade, tartar, and bearnaise sauces. Tarragon enhances fish, pork, beef, lamb, game, poultry, patés, rice, barley, vinegars, mayonnaise, and butter. It also goes well with a number of vegetables, including potatoes, tomatoes, carrots, onions, beets, asparagus, mushrooms, cauliflower, and broccoli.

Both the extract and essential oil of tarragon provide antimicrobial benefits. One of its compounds, caffeic acid, is especially effective against viruses, fungi, and bacteria. While it may not be as strongly antimicrobial as some herbs, its mildness recommends it as an herb that can be used regularly to good effect. It combats *Staphylococcus aureus* and *E. coli*, and helps curb excessive bacteria from growing in the small intestine. This antibacterial effect makes it a natural preservative for foods such as cheese. Another antibacterial compound in tarragon is eugenol. This is the substance responsible for the herb's oral anesthetic effect.

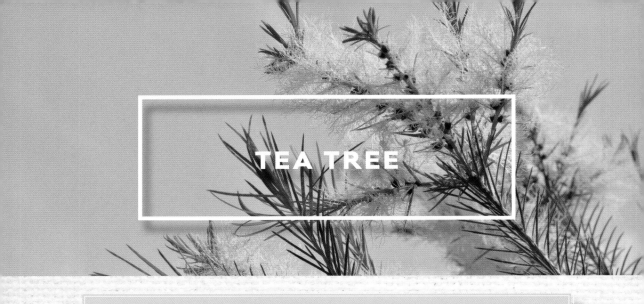

TEA TREE

BOTANICAL NAME: *MELALEUCA ALTERNIFOLIA*

On his first voyage to Australia, Captain Cook made a sharp-tasting tea from tea tree leaves and later used them in brewing beer. Eventually the leaves and then the essential oil were used to purify water. Australian soldiers and sailors used the essential oil as an all-purpose healing agent during World War II. More recently, essential oil companies have begun touting tea tree's healing properties. Medical journal articles support reports of its ability to heal mouth infections, and its primary use is in products for gum infection and canker sores, germicidal soaps, and deodorants. Tea tree essential oil is sometimes sold as Melaleuca (its botanical name)—an attempt to make it sound more exotic.

Tea tree is effective against bacteria, fungi, and viruses. It stimulates the immune system. Use it in compresses, salves, massage oil, and washes to fight all sorts of infections, including herpes, shingles, chicken pox, candida, thrush, flu, common cold, and urinary tract infections. An all-purpose wellness blend can be made from an ounce of jojoba oil, to which has been added several drops each of tea tree, bay, benzoin, geranium, hyssop, and thyme. The blend can be applied to the throat, chest, and upper back before going out for the day.

Studies show that the presence of blood and pus from infection only increase tea tree's antiseptic powers. It heals wounds, protects skin from radiation burns from cancer therapy, and encourages scar tissue to regenerate. Tea tree also treats diaper rash, acne, wounds, and insect bites. Adding just one drop to dish and diaper washing rinses gets rid of bacteria. It is one of the most non-irritating antiseptic oils, but some people do find it slightly irritating when applied topically. Those people often find an excellent alternative in tea tree's close relative, the milder niaouli.

Super-Smelling Bathroom Disinfectant

Use this all-purpose antimicrobial blend as a daily or finishing wipe on sinks, toilets, and tubs.

-20 drops tea tree oil

-10 drops basil oil

-10 drops rosemary oil

-5 drops clove oil

-5 drops eucalyptus oil

-1½ ounces distilled water

-½ ounce rubbing alcohol

Add all ingredients to a dark glass spray bottle. Shake thoroughly before each use.

Mold Destroyer

Add a teaspoon of tea tree oil, 10 drops of clove oil, and a cup of white vinegar to a spray bottle and shake thoroughly. Spray the mixture on moldy areas in the bathroom and kitchen. Leave it on for 10 or more minutes and then wipe it away. Tea tree oil can also be used as a mold preventative on tubs, toilets, and shower curtains.

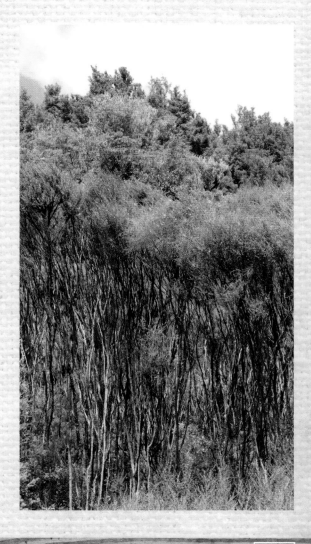

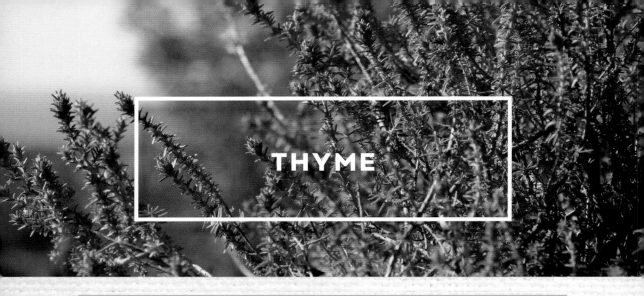

THYME

Most people consider this low-growing perennial evergreen no more than a culinary seasoning, yet its fragrance led Rudyard Kipling to write of "our close-bit thyme that smells like dawn in paradise." Thyme was used in Muslim countries for fumigating houses; frankincense was added when people could afford it. The compound thymol, derived from thyme essential oil, is one of the strongest antiseptics known and has been isolated as an ingredient in drugstore gargles, mouthwashes, cough drops, and vapor chest balms. Some of the best-known products that contain thymol are Listerine mouthwash and Vicks VapoRub. It is diluted to 0.1 percent in some natural toothpastes—and still kills the harmful microbes found in the mouth.

As an essential oil, thyme cannot be underrated. It is a superb antiseptic, with exceptional antibacterial and antifungal properties. It destroys parasitic infections as well. In fact, it acts with equal effectiveness against all four classes of pathogens. It can therefore be used— cautiously—to deal with almost all infectious health issues. It helps dissipate muscle and rheumatic pain, stops coughing, decreases gas and indigestion, stimulates menstruation, clears lung congestion, and stimulates the immune system (especially the production of white blood cells) and circulation. The essential oil is primarily used as part of a compress or sometimes in a salve or cream to fight serious infection. It is also useful for treating gum and mouth infections, such as thrush.

A Powerful Oil

Thyme essential oil can irritate the skin and mucus membranes as well as raise blood pressure, so be sure to use it only in very low dilutions. Red thyme oil is even stronger than the white and is rarely used, except in a liniment for its increased heating effects. Essential oils of thyme are sometimes available in which the most potent components, thymol and carvacrol, are removed, although this decreases their antiseptic properties. Thyme essential oil should not be used with pregnant women or children. Thyme does destroy intestinal worms, but the essential oil should not be taken internally. Instead, use the herb itself in the form of a tea or tincture.

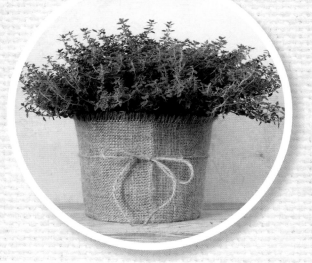

Skin Healing Blend

Diluted thyme oil is an effective skin healer. To fight skin infections and help heal wounds, make a blend of thyme and other healing essential oils with a carrier oil.

–6 drops thyme oil

–6 drops helichrysum oil

–5 drops frankincense oil

–5 drops myrrh oil

Add all oils to an ounce of fractionated coconut oil. Apply to problem area after cleaning, up to four times a day.

Thyme is not difficult to grow yourself. Harvest leaves any time for fresh use. Pick before and during flowering, and hang-dry. Alleviating a sore throat or cough can be as simple as steeping the fresh leaves in hot water for 10 minutes and drinking the tea. Thyme is an expectorant, so it can help clear mucous from congested passageways. Simply drinking a cup (or gargling with it) when you are feeling under the weather may ward off respiratory illness. Thyme tea eases other respiratory problems like allergies, sinusitis, and hay fever. It can even reduce the severity of asthma attacks. If you don't have thyme essential oil around, the tea can be used instead as a wash for skin infections, insect bites, and fungal foot issues like athlete's foot.

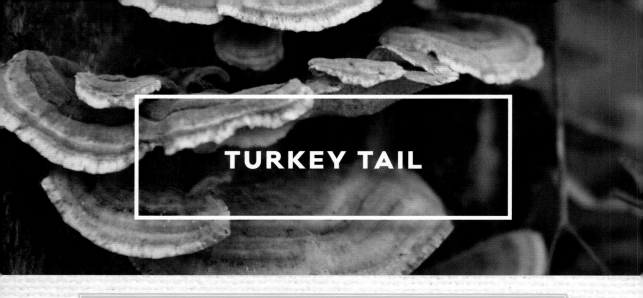

TURKEY TAIL

BOTANICAL NAME: *TRAMETES VERSICOLOR*

Turkey tail is among the most studied and understood medicinal mushrooms. While most others are lauded for what they *might* or *can* do to improve health, there is more hard evidence when it comes to the turkey tail. So much so, in fact, that one of its many beneficial compounds, *Polysaccharide K* (PSK), is an approved anti-cancer prescription drug in Asia. The Chinese have been brewing it for thousands of years as a medicinal tea. The Japanese considered it a boon to health, longevity, and spiritual attunement.

The turkey tail grows all over the world, so it's no surprise that it became popular in Europe and the Americas as well. The mushroom was used in traditional European herbal healing and by many Native American tribes. Today, it is the subject of intense study among scientists in America and all over the world due to the results of promising early tests.

Rich in many key nutrients and linked in early experiments with immunity-boosting prop-erties, turkey tail may be one of the leading medicinal mushrooms for improved overall health. A 2011 study demonstrated that it contained a unique protein called TVC that stimulated the immune system and modulated its response—keeping it from harming itself. This came as a possible breakthrough for use against autoimmune diseases like rheumatoid arthritis. Its antioxidants, immune system effects, and potential to combat inflammation make turkey tail a go-to addition to the diet of many looking to combat illnesses ranging from the common cold to chronic inflammatory dis-eases. Other evidence suggests that turkey tail might be effective for improved gastrointes-tinal health and as a possible enhancer of the liver's natural detoxification properties. There has also been research into its possible effec-tiveness in the treatment of HIV. The most news-making research attached to turkey tail, however, comes in the area of cancer research. One test tube study found that the aforemen-tioned PSK inhibited the growth and spread of human colon cancer cells. PSK has been the best-selling anticancer drug in Japan. It is used in combination with surgery, chemotherapy, and radiation therapy. The ability of PSK to regenerate necessary white blood cells and stimulate the activity and creation of cancer-killing cells has received worldwide attention.

Daily doses of Coriolus versicolor glucan (CVG), a polysaccharide found in turkey tail mushrooms, significantly reduced tumor size in a study of mice. The latter result was attributed to enhanced immune system response due to the treatments. And a rare study of the impacts of turkey tail extract on cancerous dogs showed increased survival times, along with a significant slowing in the spread of cancer cells.

One of the most thorough recent research efforts into turkey tail's cancer-fighting efficacy was concluded in 2010. The seven-year study was funded by the National Institutes of Health and carried out by researchers at the University of Minnesota and Bastyr University. They studied women with stages I-III breast cancer who had completed chemotherapy or radiation therapy. The findings were impressive, showing enhanced immune function in women who took a daily dose of turkey tail in pill form. What's more, researchers determined that the improvement was dose-dependent, and that none of the women suffered adverse side effects. The study did not identify exactly *how* the turkey tail worked for these women, but one theory holds that the mushroom improves the ability of the body's natural cancer-killing cells to do their jobs. The FDA approved this clinical trial. However, PSK has not been approved for medical use in the United States as it has been in some Asian countries.

It's not difficult to see how this medicinal mushroom got its name. Resembling the tail of the bird that produces many a Thanksgiving meal, its "plume" can be a colorful mix of browns, reds, blues, tans, and creams. *Versicolor* is Latin for many-colored.

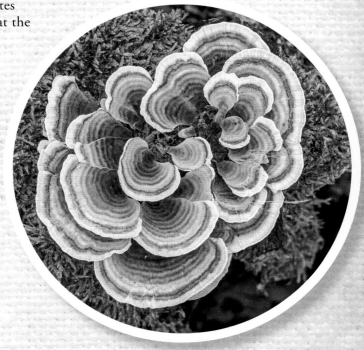

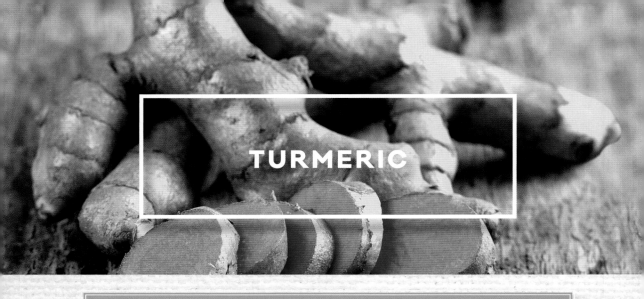

TURMERIC

BOTANICAL NAME: *CURCUMA LONGA*

Some food crops have been cultivated by humans so long that it is no longer clear when they were first domesticated or where they originated. Turmeric is one such plant. It is a sterile triploid—it produces no seeds and can't be found in the wild. Its closest relative may be *C. aromatica*, which is native to India. It seems probable that turmeric comes from southern or western India, but this has yet to be proven. A number of other wild species can be found throughout the southeastern region of Asia. It is a member of the ginger family.

Humans have been growing and harvesting turmeric for at least 4,000 years—probably longer. One of its first uses may have been as a dye for cloth. We know that the Vedic culture of India used turmeric as a culinary and medicinal spice and for religious purposes at least this long ago thanks to oral histories that made their way into the written record. Its vibrant yellow color suggested an affinity with the sun, and it was probably due to this that it became associated with sun-worshipping rituals.

In the Atharva Veda (a collection of Vedic scriptures compiled in Sanskrit roughly 3,000 years ago) turmeric makes a prominent appearance as *haridra*. Even in those ancient times, it was noted as a multipurpose panacea. A mixture of haridra powder and honey was taken to improve memory. Mixed with ghee, it was applied to snake bites. It was thought to help counteract graying hair. A significant number of remedies for skin diseases included haridra in their list of ingredients. From these origins, the root became a common ingredient in ayurvedic medicine. By 250 BC, the famous ayurvedic physician Sushruta noted in his Compendium that an ointment of turmeric would relieve food poisoning and heal wounds.

The compound that gives the plant its distinctive yellow color, curcumin, also gives it powerful healing benefits. But curcumin isn't the only molecule in turmeric with healing properties: the plant is packed with such exotic-sounding substances as sesquiterpenes, borneol, and valeric acid, to name a few.

They all work together to give turmeric its much-lauded anti-inflammatory and antioxidant qualities.

Ayurvedic healing practices used turmeric to purify the blood, treat epilepsy, ease diarrhea, treat respiratory ailments, fight infection, and treat urinary tract issues. It was used as a paste, dried powder, and in juice form. The ayurvedic system considers turmeric to be a balancing agent that helps the human system achieve harmony among the three doshas. It continues to play a role in ayurvedic healing.

Turmeric Essential Oil

As an inexpensive and widely available essential oil, turmeric is a must-have for your medicine cabinet. Turmeric oil is especially prized for its anti-inflammatory properties, making it a great choice for soothing arthritis, muscle pain, headaches, and gastrointestinal inflammation. A few drops in a carrier oil applied to the skin can improve elasticity and reduce wrinkles, thanks to turmeric's antioxidant effects. When ingested in small quantities, turmeric oil helps to ward off infection and support the body's immune defenses. And research shows that turmeric can improve metabolic function in diabetics, as well as boost heart health.

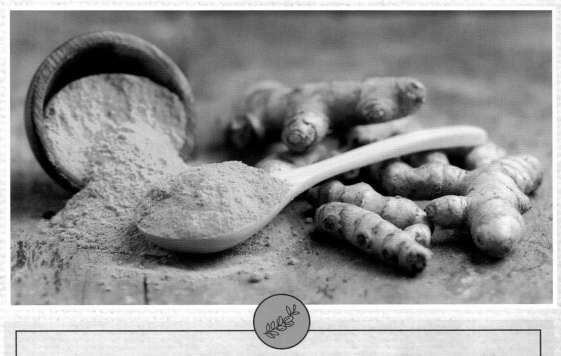

Vivid orange turmeric powder contributes to curry powder's distinctive color and gives the spice an added layer of complexity.

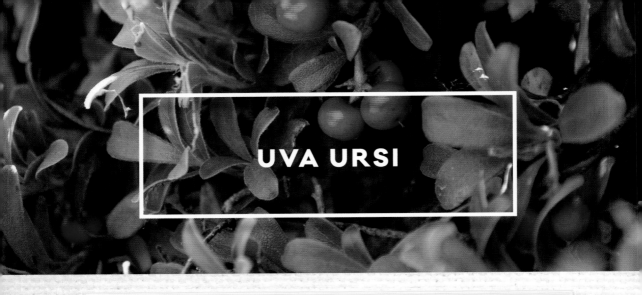

UVA URSI

BOTANICAL NAME: *ARCTOSTAPHYLOS UVA URSI*

Uva ursi, sometimes called bearberry or kinni-kinnick, has leaves containing up to 40 percent tannic acid, enough to make them once useful in tanning leather. Tannins and the glycoside arbutin give uva ursi its astringent and antiseptic properties. Native Americans used uva ursi as a remedy for urinary tract infections.

Herbalists suggest uva ursi primarily to treat bladder issues. Uva ursi is particularly indicated for illnesses caused by *E. coli*, a bacterium that lives in the intestines and can invade the urinary tract. It works particularly well in the alkaline environment this bacteria produces. That said, care must be taken when using uva ursi, as it displays some toxicity and may irritate the liver if used too long or in too high a dose. Externally, the herb has been used to treat sprains, swellings, and sore muscles. A salve can be made from the berries for topical application. This can be directly applied to burns, canker sores, bruises, wounds, and inflamed areas. The acids in the salve help accelerate healing while reducing inflammation.

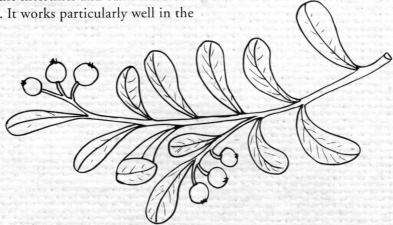

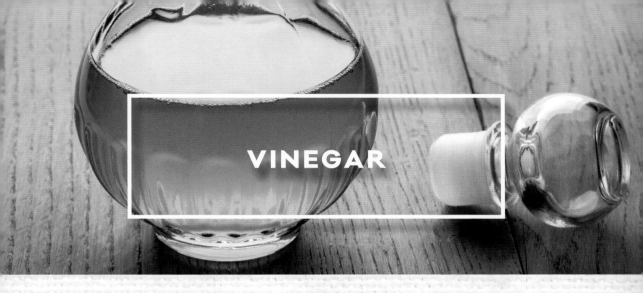

VINEGAR

Vinegar has been valued for its healing properties for a long time. It has found its way from the apothecary's shelf to the cook's pot. There seems hardly an ailment that vinegar has not been touted to cure at some point in history. While science has yet to prove the effectiveness of many of these cures, scores of people still praise vinegar as a healthful and healing food.

Today, it can continue to play that dual role, taking the place of less healthful dietary ingredients and helping to regulate blood sugar levels while entertaining our taste buds with its tart flavor. Fans view vinegar as an overall health-boosting tonic and recommend mixing a teaspoon or tablespoon of cider vinegar with a glass of water and drinking it each morning or before meals. (Apple cider vinegar is the traditional vinegar of choice for home or folk remedies, although some recent claims have been made for the benefits of wine vinegars, especially red wine vinegar.)

Those who have faith in apple cider vinegar as a wide-ranging cure say its healing properties come from an abundance of nutrients that remain after apples are fermented to make apple cider vinegar. They contend that vinegar is rich in minerals and vitamins, including calcium, potassium, and beta carotene; complex carbohydrates and fiber, including the soluble fiber pectin; amino acids (the building blocks of protein); beneficial enzymes; and acetic acid (which gives vinegar its taste).

These substances do play many important roles in health and healing, and some are even considered essential nutrients for human health. The problem is that standard nutritional analysis of vinegar, including apple cider vinegar, has yet to show it to be a good source of most of these substances.

How Can Vinegar Help?

So if vinegar doesn't actually contain all the substances that are supposed to account for its medicinal benefits, does that mean it has no healing powers? Hardly. We can't totally rule out many of the dramatic claims made for it. Although we know vinegar doesn't contain loads of nutrients traditionally associated with good health, it may well contain yet-to-be-identified phytochemicals that would account for some of the healing benefits that vinegar fans swear by. Scientists continue to discover such beneficial substances in all kinds of foods.

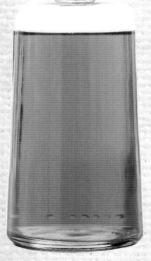

But beyond that possibility, there appear to be more tangible and realistic—albeit less sensational—ways that vinegar can help the body keep itself healthy. Rather than being the dramatic blockbuster cure that we are endlessly (and probably fruitlessly) searching for, vinegar seems quite capable of playing myriad supporting roles—as part of an overall lifestyle approach—that can indeed help us fight serious health conditions, such as osteoporosis, diabetes, and heart disease.

Increasing Calcium Absorption

If there is one thing vinegar fans, marketers, alternative therapists, and scientists alike can agree on, it's that vinegar is high in acetic acid. And acetic acid, like other acids, can increase the body's absorption of important minerals from the foods we eat. Therefore, including apple cider vinegar in meals or possibly even drinking a mild tonic of vinegar and water (up to a tablespoon in a glass of water) just before or with meals might improve your body's ability to absorb the essential minerals locked in foods.

Vinegar may be especially useful to women, who generally have a hard time getting all the calcium their bodies need to keep bones strong and prevent the debilitating, bone-thinning disease osteoporosis. Although dietary calcium is most abundant in dairy products such as milk, many women (and men) suffer from a condition called lactose intolerance that makes it difficult or impossible for them to digest the sugar in milk. As a result, they may suffer uncomfortable gastrointestinal symptoms, such as cramping and diarrhea, when they consume dairy products. These women must often look elsewhere to fulfill their dietary calcium needs.

Dark, leafy greens are good sources of calcium, but some of these greens also contain compounds that inhibit calcium absorption. Fortunately for dairy-deprived women (and even those who do drink milk), a few splashes of vinegar or a tangy vinaigrette on their greens may very well allow them to absorb more valuable calcium. Don't you wish all medications were so tasty?

Making a Healthy Diet Easier to Swallow

Some of our strongest natural weapons against cancer and aging are fruits and vegetables. Their antioxidants also help to protect cells from the free-radical damage that is thought to underlie many of the changes we associate with aging. Protected cells don't wear out and need replacing as often as cells that aren't bathed in antioxidants. Scientists think this continual cell replacement may be at the root of aging.

We're supposed to eat several cups of fruits as well as vegetables per day. One way to add excitement and variety to all those vegetables is to use vinegar liberally as a seasoning.

• Rice vinegar and a little soy sauce give veggies an Asian flavor or can form the base of an Asian coleslaw.

• Red wine vinegar or white wine vinegar can turn boring vegetables into a quick-and-easy marinated-vegetable salad that's ready to grab out of the refrigerator whenever hunger strikes. Just chop your favorite veggies, put them in a bowl with a marinade of vintegar, herbs, and a dash of olive oil, and let them sit for at least an hour.

• Toss chopped vegetables in a vinegar-and-olive-oil salad dressing before loading them on skewers and putting them on the backyard grill. The aroma and flavor will actually have your family asking for seconds.

• After steaming vegetables, drizzle a little of your favorite vinegar over them instead of adding butter or salt. They'll taste so good, you may never get to the meat on your plate.

Washing produce in a mixture of water and vinegar appears to help remove certain pesticides, according to the small amount of research that has been published. Vinegar also appears to be helpful in getting rid of harmful bacteria on fruits and vegetables. To help remove potentially harmful residues, mix a solution of 10 percent vinegar to 90 percent water (for example, mix one cup of white vinegar in nine cups of water). Then, place the produce in the vinegar solution, let it soak briefly, and then swish it around in the solution. Finally, rinse the produce thoroughly.

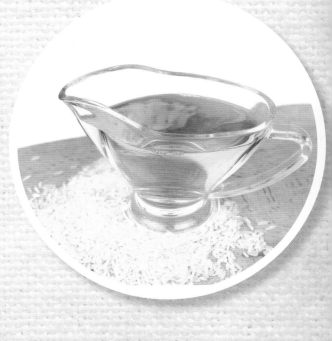

Remedies for Minor Ailments

Vinegar's potential for treating or preventing major medical problems is of interest to almost everyone. But it also has been cherished as a home remedy for some common minor ailments for centuries. Although they're not life-or-death issues, these minor health problems can be uncomfortable, and there is often little modern medicine can offer in the way of a cure. So you may want to give vinegar a shot to determine for yourself if it can help.

Apple cider vinegar is the second-most-common type of vinegar in the United States. This light-tan vinegar made from apple cider adds a tart and subtle fruity flavor to your cooking. Apple cider vinegar is the preferred go-to vinegar to use when creating homemade vinegar-based remedies.

Stomach upset: To settle minor stomach upset, try a simple cider vinegar tonic with a meal. Drinking a mixture of a spoonful of vinegar in a glass of water is said to improve digestion and ease minor stomach upset by stimulating digestive juices.

Common cold symptoms: Apple cider vinegar is also an age-old treatment for symptoms of the common cold. For a sore throat, mix one teaspoon of apple cider vinegar into a glass of water; gargle with a mouthful of the solution and then swallow it, repeating until you've finished all the solution in the glass. For a natural cough syrup, mix half a tablespoon apple cider vinegar with half a tablespoon honey and swallow. Finally, you can add a quarter-cup of apple cider vinegar to the recommended amount of water in your room vaporizer to help with congestion.

Itching or stinging from minor insect bites: In the folklore of New England, rural Indiana, and parts of the Southwest, a vinegar wash is sometimes used for treating bites and stings. (However, if the person bitten has a known allergy to insect venom or begins to exhibit signs of a serious allergic reaction, such as widespread hives, swelling of the face or mouth, difficulty breathing, or loss of consciousness, skip the home remedies and seek immediate medical attention.) Pour undiluted vinegar over the bite or sting, avoiding surrounding healthy skin as much as possible

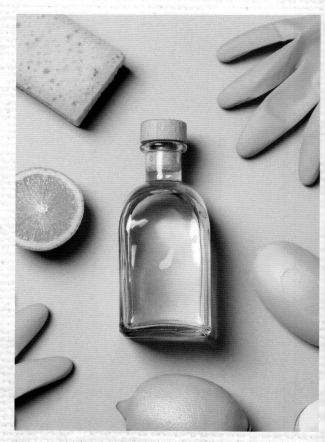

Poison Ivy

Contact with poison ivy, poison oak, or poison sumac often goes hand-in-hand with camping and other outdoor activities. Outdoor enthusiasts by the tentful have had to cut trips short after an unfortunate encounter. The problem stems from the colorless oil called urushiol. Whenever one of these plants is cut, crushed, stepped on, sat on, grabbed, or disturbed, the oil is released. Once on the victim, the toxic oil penetrates the skin and a rash appears within 12 to 48 hours after exposure. Since poison plant oils don't just disappear, it's crucial to wash anything that has had contact with the victim or the oil.

Allergic reactions from these plants, along with other allergic skin reactions, can be tamed by a simple vinegar rinse. First wash the affected area with soap and lukewarm water, then rinse. Apply vinegar with a cotton ball, rub gently, and rinse. Before going to bed, pour a cup of baking soda into a lukewarm bath and take a soak. A vinegar rinse is also helpful in easing the pain of sunburn.

Acne

Use a clean travel-size bottle to mix 1 teaspoon vinegar and 10 teaspoons water. Clean your face as usual in the morning, then carry this bottle and a few cotton balls with you so you can dab acne spots several times during the day. This solution shouldn't dry out your skin, and the vinegar will help return your skin to a natural pH balance. The treatment may also help prevent future acne outbreaks. Discontinue use if irritation worsens.

Make a paste of honey, wheat flour, and vinegar, then use it to lightly cover a new outbreak of pimples. Keep paste on overnight, and rinse off in the morning. This should enhance the healing process.

Dandruff

Vinegar is a great hair conditioner and can improve cleanliness and shine. For simple conditioning, just add 1 tablespoon vinegar to your hair as you rinse it.

To control problem dandruff, mix 2 cups water and ½ cup vinegar, and use this as a rinse after shampooing. If you need an even stronger treatment for dandruff control, use this same method, but keep the rinse on your hair for an hour, covered with a shower cap. Rinse. This mixture will also help control frizziness in dry or damaged hair.

Vinegar can even help control an infestation of head lice. First use a medicated head lice shampoo, or follow your doctor's instructions for lice control. After shampooing hair, rinse with white vinegar, and go through hair with a fine comb dipped in vinegar. The vinegar will help to loosen any remaining nits, or eggs, from hair. Continue with treatment prescribed on shampoo bottle.

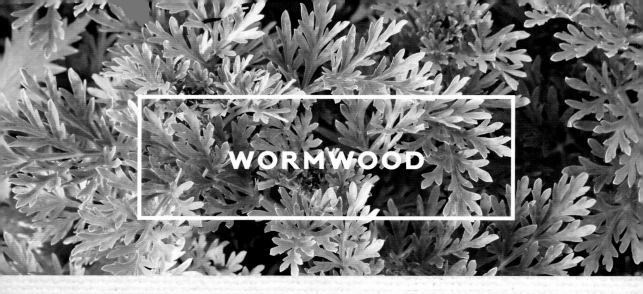

WORMWOOD

BOTANICAL NAME: *ARTEMISIA ABSINTHIUM*

Wormwood is steeped in mystique. It is said to have grown up in the trail left by the serpent as it slithered from the Garden of Eden. In ancient Egypt, it was used as a medicinal plant for anal pain and as an additive to wine. In Europe, the herb became the prime ingredient of the addictive alcoholic drink called absinthe, which is illegal in most countries, including the United States. Wormwood got its name because it expels intestinal worms. It is especially effective at eliminating pinworms and roundworms. Caution must be used when taking wormwood internally, but when used correctly, it provides relief for symptoms of Crohn's disease as well as small intestine bacterial overgrowth. The plant also is an antiseptic, antispasmodic, and carminative, and it increases bile production. It has been used to treat fever, colds, jaundice, and gallstones.

Compresses soaked in the tea are said to be good for irritations, bruises, and sprains. Wormwood oil has been used as a liniment to relieve the pain of rheumatism, neuralgia, and arthritis. The plant is also a broad-spectrum antifungal and antibacterial, and research indicates that compounds in one of the species of wormwood, *A. annua*, could be a cure for malaria. Wormwood is also a flea and moth repellant. Although it is brittle when dried, it makes a beautiful foundation for a wreath or swag.

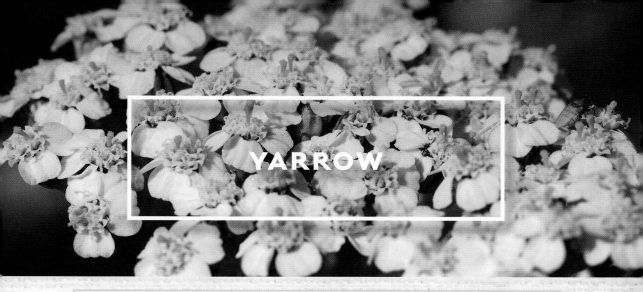

YARROW

BOTANICAL NAME: *ACHILLEA MILLEFOLIUM*

In the epic *Iliad*, Homer reports that legendary warrior Achilles used yarrow leaves to treat the wounds of his fallen comrades. Studies show that yarrow is a fine herb indeed for accelerating healing of cuts and bruises. The Greeks used the herb to stop hemorrhages. Gerard's famous herbal cited yarrow's benefits in 1597. And after colonists brought the plant to America, Indians used it to treat bleeding, wounds, infections, headaches, indigestion, and sore throat.

Clinical studies have supported the longstanding use of yarrow to cleanse wounds and make blood clot faster. Yarrow treats bleeding stomach ulcers, heavy menstrual periods, and bleeding from the bowels. An essential oil known as azulene is responsible for yarrow's ability to reduce inflammation. In traditional Chinese medicine, yarrow is credited with the ability to nurture the spleen, liver, kidney, and bladder. Several studies have shown that yarrow improves uterine tone and reduces uterine spasms in animals. Apigenin and flavonoid constituents are credited with yarrow's antispasmodic properties. The herb also contains salicylic acid, aspirin's main constituent, making it useful for relieving pain. Chewing the leaves or root is an old toothache remedy.

Yarrow fights bacteria and dries up congestion in sinus and other respiratory infections and allergies. The plant has long been a standby herb for promoting sweating to bring down fevers in cases of colds and influenza. It also relieves bladder infections. Because of its astringent and cleansing properties, yarrow is sometimes added to skin lotions.

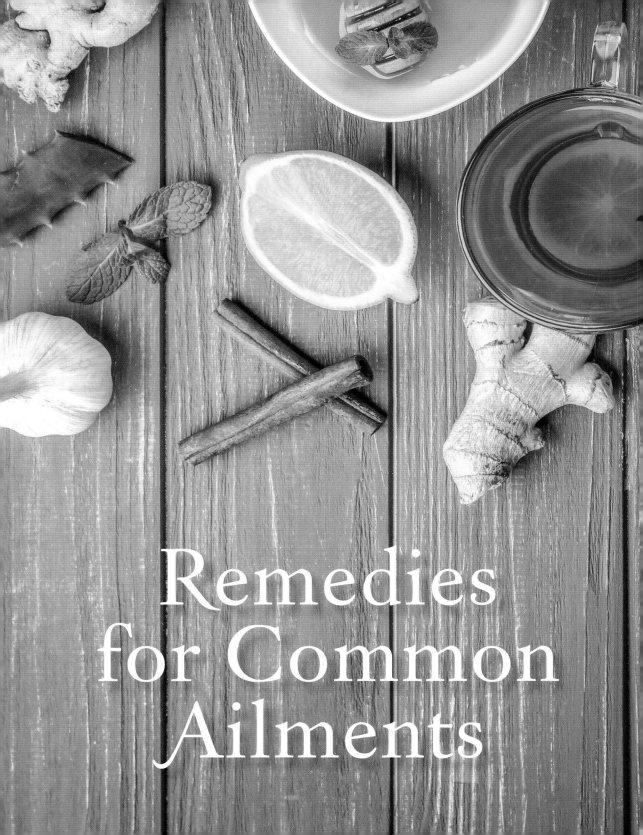

Remedies
for Common
Ailments

Can effective antimicrobial weapons against today's superbugs be found in dusty ancient manuscripts? Apparently, yes. In 2015, researchers at the University of Nottingham, England, conducted an experiment that resulted in an amazing discovery.

Bald's Leechbook, a medical text from 10th-century England, contains an eye salve recipe for styes (infected eyelash follicles). The researchers recreated the salve to test against various pathogens. The recipe contained ingredients with known antibiotic properties (garlic, wine, and onions or leeks) but also called for "oxgall" (cow's bile). The recipe specifically noted that the mixture must be prepared in a brass vessel and allowed to sit undisturbed for nine days. These instructions were carefully followed. They then tested the remedy against biofilms and infected mouse tissue containing the infamous methicillin-resistant *Staphylococcus aureus* (MRSA). The recipe almost completely wiped out the bacteria. In fact, it performed better than vancomycin, one of the last-ditch medicines used against the superbug.

The researchers noted that individual components of the recipe did not perform as well against the staph. Instead, there seemed to be a synergy between these components which led to the impressive results. This suggests that fairly sophisticated procedural practices were in place during a period not typically thought of as medically advanced. It also reminds us that the practice of combining natural compounds for healing was one of the traditions modern medicine grew from. What other simple combinations of natural ingredients await our discovery? Or rediscovery?

The remedies for common ailments in the following pages don't come from dusty manuscripts, but they are the kind of time-tested, pragmatic cures that have stuck around because of their efficacy. They are simple to use, effective, and affordable. Herbs, teas, and essential oils are more readily available today than ever before. If you don't find it in your local grocery or health food store, you can probably find it online. This chapter will help you use those healing compounds to best effect.

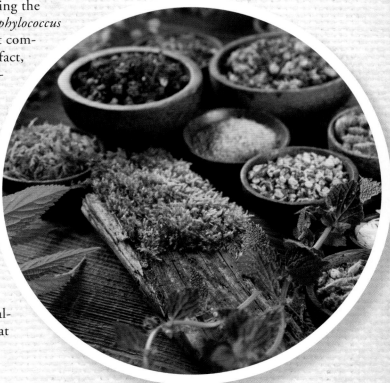

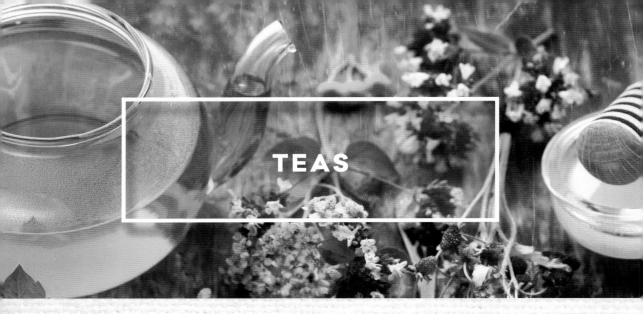

TEAS

One of the easiest and most popular ways of preparing an herbal medicine is to brew a tea. There are two types of teas: infusions and decoctions. An infusion is simply the result of steeping herbs in hot water. A decoction is the result of boiling herbs gently in water. When you simmer cinnamon sticks and cloves in apple cider, you're making a decoction.

In general, delicate leaves and flowers are best infused; boiling may cause them to lose the volatile essential oils. Infusions use around 1 teaspoon of dried herbs per 1 cup of hot water. (If you use fresh herbs, use 1 to 2 teaspoons or more). Pour the hot water over the herbs in a pan or teapot, cover with a lid, and allow to steep for about ten minutes. Strain and drink. Finely cut herbs in tea bags steep much faster—in about five minutes. To make larger quantities of hot infusions, use 5 tablespoons of herbs per gallon of water.

Extremely volatile herbs such as peppermint and lemon balm lose a lot of essential oils with high heat. These herbs can be infused with cold water. It is easy to recognize volatile herbs because they are highly fragrant. Allow a cold tea to infuse overnight. These herbs are suitable for making the popular "sun" tea. Using 1 teaspoon of herbs per cup of water, put herbs and water in a jar, and place in the sun for a couple of hours.

Roots, barks, and seeds, on the other hand, are best made into decoctions because these hard, woody materials need significant boiling time to get the constituents out of the fiber. Fresh roots generally should be sliced thin. To prepare a medicinal decoction, use one teaspoon of herbs per cup of water, cover, and gently simmer for 15 to 30 minutes. Strain the decoction. Use glass, ceramic, or earthenware pots to make your decoction—aluminum may taint herbal teas. A tea will remain fresh for several days in the refrigerator. To preserve teas, make a concentrated brew, three times as strong as an ordinary remedy. Then add one part of drinking alcohol (not rubbing alcohol) to 3 parts of the infusion. Store in covered container. When ready to use, dilute with 3 parts water. How much of an infusion or decoction should you take at one time? In general, drink 1 cup three times a day.

Lemon Mint Tea

A simple tea to make, this remedy is excellent for colds.

- ¼ cup dried peppermint leaves
- ⅓ cup dried lemon balm leaves
- 3 tablespoons dried organic lemon rind, grated or diced

Combine ingredients. Bring a cup of water to a boil. Remove from heat, and steep 1 to 2 tablespoons of the herb mixture in the water for 15 minutes; strain and drink. This tea is delicious either hot or iced.

Stomach Relief Tea

Here's a remedy that can quiet stomach discomfort, from indigestion to a spastic colon.

- 1 tablespoon dried chamomile flowers
- 1 teaspoon fennel seeds
- 2 tablespoon dried mint leaves

Combine ingredients. Steep 1 teaspoon of the mixture in a cup of hot water for 15 minutes; strain and drink.

Traveler's Tea

Holidays and vacations that feature airport terminals, crowded trains, busy restaurants, and bustling hotels can dramatically increase your exposure to all kinds of tenacious and exotic pathogens. Rest and hydration will give you a good start, but how can you keep yourself from getting sick once you're on the road? Try bringing along a supply of this immunity-boosting blend. The tart and fruity ingredients give it an invigorating zing that you won't mind sipping hot or cold.

- 2 tablespoons green tea
- 1 tablespoon dried elderberries
- 1 tablespoon dried hibiscus
- 1 tablespoon dried lemongrass
- ½ tablespoon dried organic lemon peel
- ½ tablespoon dried rose hips

Mix all ingredients and store in an airtight container. Steep 1–2 teaspoons of the mixture in a cup of hot water for 15 minutes; strain and drink. This blend can be enhanced with dried ginger pieces, whole black peppercorns, cloves, or echinacea.

Take a Deep Breath and Reset Tea

Back home and a bit frazzled from your travels? Picked up a cough along the way? Have this on hand and ready to brew when you finally arrive home. This earthy, replenishing blend is an all-purpose restorative that will bring you back to balance and ground you in calmness. It is also an excellent blend for the depths of winter, with warm and spicy notes to keep out the gloom. You must have chaga tea already on hand to prepare this recipe.

–16 ounces chaga tea
–1 teaspoon lightly crushed fenugreek seeds
–½ teaspoon dried elecampane root pieces
–1 small slice fresh ginger

Warm the tea over low heat and add the dry ingredients, giving them time to simmer (do not boil) and release into the liquid, a minimum of 30 minutes. Chaga tea which has been prepared properly will already have a small amount of aromatic vanillic acid in it. You can bring this note out further by adding a sliver of vanilla bean to the brew. About 15 minutes before removing from heat, add the following:

–1 or 2 dried allspice berries
–1 or 2 slivers of cinnamon stick
–1 whole clove

Strain and drink.

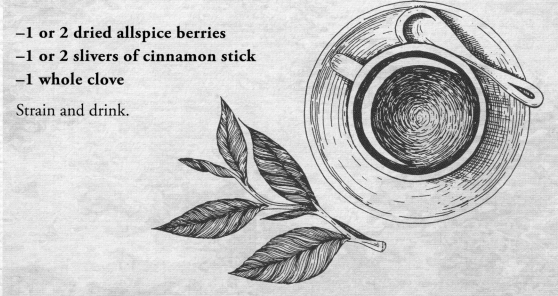

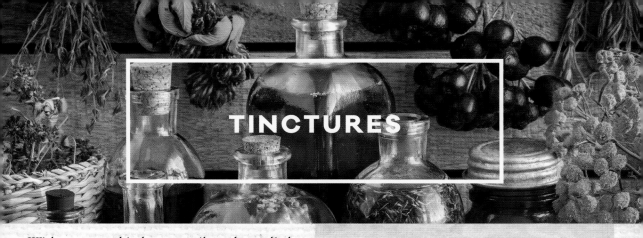

TINCTURES

With common kitchen utensils and very little effort, you can easily prepare suitable tinctures for your own use. First, clean and pick over dried or fresh herbs, removing any insects or damaged plant material. Remove leaves and flowers from stems. Cut the plant parts you want to process into small pieces, or chop them in a blender or food processor. Cover with just enough drinking alcohol to completely submerge the herbs. The spirit most commonly used is 80 to 100 proof vodka. Some herbs, such as ginger and cayenne, require the higher alcohol content to fully extract their constituents.

Puree the material and transfer it to a glass jar. After it settles, make certain the alcohol covers the plants. This is especially important if you use fresh herbs. Plant materials exposed to air can mold or rot. Store the jar at room temperature out of sunlight, and shake the jar every day. After two weeks, strain through a cheesecloth, thin piece of muslin, or paper coffee filter. If particles eventually settle after the tincture has been stored, shake the mixture to redistribute them. Tinctures will keep for many years without refrigeration.

Simple Dandelion Tincture

Try out this simple recipe—all it involves is dandelion roots and vodka. Place dried, chopped dandelion roots in a food processor with enough 80 to 100 proof vodka to process. Once blended, store in a glass jar, shake daily, and strain in two weeks. Take ½ to 1 teaspoon three times a day before meals for chronic constipation, poor digestion, or urinary tract problems, or as a spring tonic.

Because the usual dose of a tincture is 30 drops, you receive enough herb to benefit from its medicinal properties with very little alcohol. If you're allergic to alcohol—or simply don't wish to use it—try making vinegar- or glycerine-based tinctures. Vinegar and glycerine dissolve plant constituents almost as effectively as spirits. Glycerine is available at most pharmacies

Vinegar Tinctures

Vinegar, which contains the solvent acetic acid, is an alternative to alcohol tinctures. You can use herbal vinegars medicinally or dilute them with more vinegar to make great-tasting salad dressings and marinades. Use any vinegar, such as apple cider, rice vinegar, red wine vinegar, or balsamic vinegar. Vinegar is also a potent antifungal agent and makes a good athlete's foot soak when combined with antimicrobial herbs.

Four Thieves Vinegar

Here's a recipe handed down from the Middle Ages. Herbal lore has it that four men caught ransacking empty homes infested with bubonic plague were tried before a court in Marseilles. Asked by the judge how they had avoided contracting the plague, the men said they had washed themselves with a special herbal vinegar. The thieves were granted freedom in return for the recipe. You can add this vinegar to a bath, or take 1 teaspoon internally—no more than 1 tablespoon an hour—to protect yourself during flu season.

–2 tablespoons **lavender**
–2 tablespoons **rosemary**
–2 tablespoons **sage**
–2 tablespoons **wormwood**
–2 tablespoons **rue**
–2 tablespoons **mint**
–2 tablespoons **garlic buds, unpeeled**

Cover the herbs with vinegar. Keep at room temperature for two weeks. Strain and bottle. You can also make a vinegar syrup by adding 4 ounces of glycerine. Sweeten to taste.

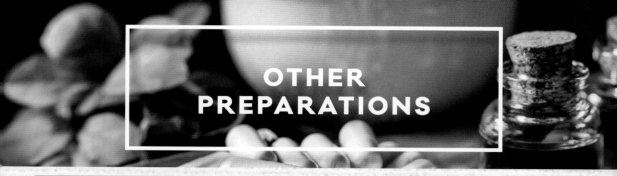

OTHER PREPARATIONS

Glycerine Tinctures

The advantage of using a glycerine-based tincture is that it does not contain alcohol. The disadvantage is that glycerine doesn't dissolve an herb's constituents as well as alcohol does. To make a glycerine tincture, mix 4 ounces water and 6 ounces glycerine. Pour the mixture over 1 ounce of dried or fresh chopped herbs in a clean jar. As with alcohol tinctures, make sure the herbs are submerged under the glycerine and water mixture. Shake daily. Let stand at room temperature for two weeks, then strain and bottle.

Pills and Capsules

We have come to rely on pharmaceutical pills to cure many of our ailments. There is nothing inherently wrong with taking pills. But if you're uncomfortable with the notion of ingesting synthetic chemicals, you can turn to herbal capsules, tablets, or lozenges. Capsules and tablets provide a convenient method of ingesting herbs that have strong, harsh flavors.

You can find empty gelatin capsules at health food stores, online herbal houses, and some pharmacies. Fill the capsules with powdered herbs. Remember, it's best to store your herbs whole, then powder them immediately before encapsulating them. You can powder them with a mortar and pestle or in a coffee grinder or food processor. If the method you use does not produce a fine powder, strain the herbs through a sieve or strainer first.

Fill half the capsule with the powdered herb and pack tightly. A chopstick is a good tool for packing the powder into the capsule. Close with the other capsule half. Many natural food stores also sell capsule makers that speed up the process.

To make herb pills, simply blend powdered herbs with a bit of honey to bind the mixture. Then just pinch off bits of the resulting sticky substance and roll into balls. (If the balls seem too moist, roll them in a mixture of slippery elm and licorice powder to soak up excess moisture.) Dry the herbal pills in a dehydrator, an oven set to preheat, or outdoors on a warm day covered with a cloth. Store the dried pills in an airtight container.

Syrups

In syrup form, even the most bitter herbs taste good. Syrups are ideal for soothing sore throats and respiratory ailments. You can make herbal syrups by combining sugar, honey, or glycerine with infusions, decoctions, tinctures, herbal juices, or medicinal liquors. Preserve syrups by refrigerating or adding glycerine. Make syrups in small quantities. To make a simple syrup, dissolve the sweetener of your choice in a hot herb infusion. You can add herbal tinctures to increase the syrup's medicinal value.

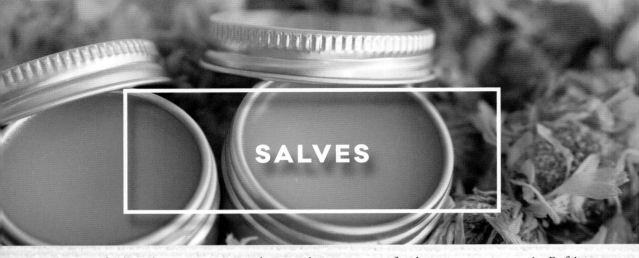

SALVES

Salves are fat-based preparations used to soothe abrasions, heal wounds and lacerations, protect babies' skin from diaper rash, and soften rough skin and chapped lips. Salves are made by heating herbs with fat or oil until the fat absorbs the plant's healing properties. Beeswax is then added to the strained mixture to give it a thicker consistency.

Kept in a cool place, salves last at least a year. You can preserve a salve even longer by adding a few drops of tincture of benzoin, poplar bud tincture, or glycerine. Make salves in small batches to keep them fresh. Store in tightly lidded jars.

The key ingredient of salves is herbal oil. Make your oil out of the herb of your choice. Calendula oil is a good base for wonderful all-purpose healing salves. St. John's wort can be used to treat swelling and bruising in traumatic injuries. Garlic oil can be used to prepare a salve to treat infectious conditions. To turn the oil into a salve, melt ¾ ounce beeswax in 1 cup herbal oil.

You can purchase beeswax from health food stores, beekeeping supply stores, and a variety of websites. Grated beeswax melts faster; use a grater or food processor to grate it. Refrigerate the wax before grating to make the job easier. (Wash utensils with very hot water to remove all the beeswax.)

Warm the herbal oil, then add the beeswax. When the beeswax melts, pour the salve into containers before the blend starts to harden. If you wish, add 500 IU of vitamin E per ounce to increase the salve's healing properties and help preserve the salve, or add a teaspoon of benzoin or poplar tincture for every cup of herbal oil to help preserve it. Other possible additives are 1 to 2 tablespoons of cocoa butter to make the consistency more creamy or ½ to 1 teaspoon hydrous lanolin per cup of herbal oil to give the salve more tack. Lanolin is especially good in a salve for diaper rash.

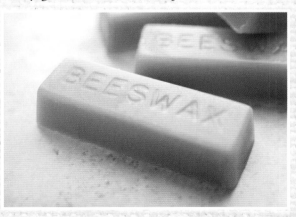

All-Purpose Healing Salve

-½ cup comfrey root oil
-½ cup calendula oil
-¾ ounce beeswax
-1 tablespoon vitamin E oil
-20 drops vitamin A emulsion

Combine the oils and gently warm them. Melt the beeswax into the oils. Add vitamins E and A. Pour into salve containers and let stand about 20 minutes to harden.

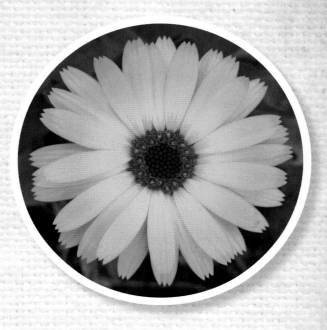

Juniper Berry Ointment

This ointment is good for wounds, itching, and scratches.

-1 cup juniper berries
-2 cups oil (olive, peanut, wheat germ, or lanolin)
-2–3 tablespoons beeswax

Simmer berries in oil. Melt beeswax into the oil and berry mixture. Strain and pour into jars.

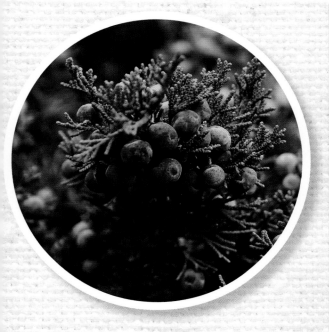

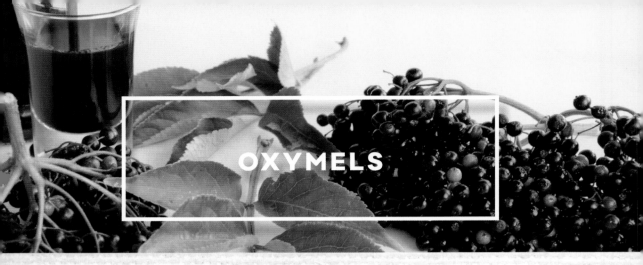

OXYMELS

An oxymel (from the Latin words denoting *acid* and *honey*) is a simple medicinal concoction with roots going back at least to the ancient Greeks. The liquid base is vinegar. Various plants are added, and the mixture is steeped for a time, allowing the vinegar to draw out the virtues of the plants. After this, the mixture is strained and honey is added. Oxymels may be taken straight (usually in amounts measured by the tablespoon or less), diluted in water, or even added to foods. In fact, an oxymel can be the exotic ingredient that takes a vinaigrette to the next level.

Oxymels work as all-purpose tonics, but they can also be crafted to address specific ailments. As your knowledge of the different properties of herbs grows, you will be able to create your own custom blends for specific purposes.

The following recipes give an idea of what can be done with oxymels. NOTE: never use metal lids when making your own oxymels. The vinegar is corrosive.

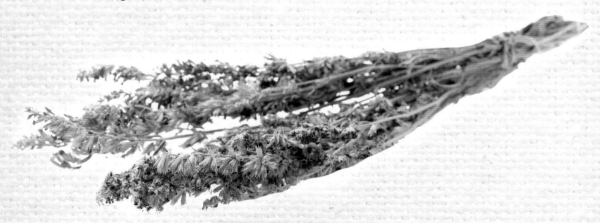

Breathe Easy Oxymel

This oxymel is good for residual congestion and lingering coughs that just won't go away after an illness. The hyssop, as noted earlier, has antispasmodic properties that make it a great choice for calming coughs—especially the kind that keep you up at night.

–⅛ cup dried hyssop
–⅛ cup dried sage
–⅛ cup dried thyme
–Raw apple cider vinegar
–Raw honey to taste

Place all herbs in a pint glass jar (wide-mouth canning jars work well). Fill jar with enough vinegar so that it is at least half full. Make sure that herbs are mixed in well. Cover with a tight-fitting (non-metal) lid. Place jar in cupboard for at least four weeks (preferably longer). Strain well and add honey to desired sweetness. Store in a dark cupboard. For coughs, take a teaspoon at a time as needed (about once an hour, especially near bedtime).

Elderberry Oxymel

Antiviral elderberry combined with ginger and elecampane make another oxymel great for vanquishing respiratory ailments. The elecampane, as noted earlier, is an expectorant. It eases shortness of breath and bronchial problems. Once this oxymel has finished steeping and has been decanted into a clear glass jar, it makes a beautiful purple liquid that looks the part of a healing elixir.

–Dried elderberries
–2–3 tablespoons dried ginger
–2–3 tablespoons elecampane root
–Raw apple cider vinegar
–Raw honey

Pour elderberries into a quart glass jar until it is at least ⅓ full. Add the ginger and elecampane. Add equal amounts vinegar and honey until mixture is covered. Mix well. Cover with a tight-fitting (non-metal) lid. The next day add more vinegar if necessary, as the dried elderberries will swell. Place jar in cupboard for at least four weeks (preferably longer). Strain well and store in the refrigerator. Use within six months.

Fire Cider

One famous all-purpose oxymel is fire cider. The recipe is credited to renowned American herbalist Rosemary Gladstar. Typically used to ward off colds and the flu during the winter months, this oxymel mobilizes your immune system and provides it with a complex arsenal of anti-inflammatory, antiviral, antibacterial, circulation-boosting compounds.

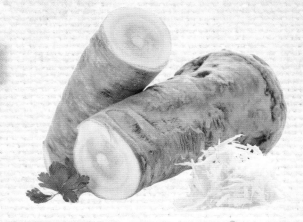

The core ingredients in fire cider include:

- Horseradish
- Ginger
- Garlic
- Onion
- Chilis (cayenne powder or fresh chili peppers)
- Raw apple cider vinegar
- Raw honey

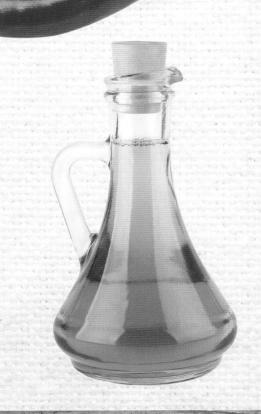

If you're using these ingredients, you're making basic fire cider. But the recipe is flexible. From the core list, feel free to add other medicinal herbs, roots, spices, and fruits. Common additions include turmeric (powder or root), echinacea, citrus fruits (especially lemon), cinnamon, cloves, and black pepper. When fresh herbs are used, common types include rosemary, oregano, thyme, and sage. When fresh chili peppers are used, common varieties include serrano, jalapeno, and habanero.

All-Purpose Fiery Oxymel

- −½ cup peeled and chopped horseradish
- −½ cup chopped onion
- −¼ cup peeled and sliced ginger
- −6 cloves garlic, peeled and crushed
- −1 jalapeno pepper, sliced
- −1 lemon, sliced
- −1 large sprig fresh rosemary
- −1 tablespoon black peppercorns
- −1 tablespoon turmeric powder
- −¼ teaspoon cayenne powder
- −Raw apple cider vinegar
- −Raw honey to taste

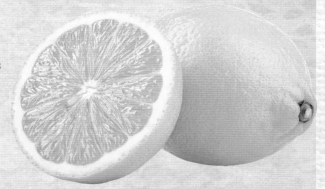

Place all ingredients (except vinegar and honey) in a quart or half-gallon glass jar. Cover with enough vinegar to cover contents by about two inches. Cover with a tight-fitting (non-metal) lid. Place jar in cupboard for at least four weeks (preferably longer). Shake the mixture once a day to help the maceration process. When ready, strain the liquid through a cheesecloth into a large mixing container. Add honey and stir thoroughly. Store the liquid in a glass bottle with a tight-fitting (non-metal) lid. Keep the bottle in a dark cupboard.

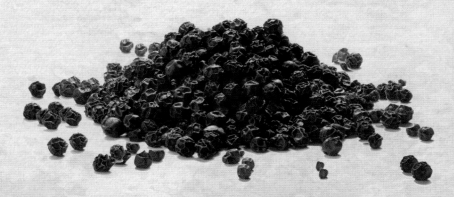

Kitchen Cupboard Immunity Oxymel

This oxymel emphasizes common kitchen herbs and spices that happen to be pathogen-beating all-stars. Use it generously at the start of cold and flu season to give your body an immunity boost. The flavor is food-friendly and fantastic—you'll naturally find all kinds of uses for it.

-1 small sliced onion
-½ cup peeled and sliced ginger
-6 whole peeled garlic cloves
-1 sprig fresh oregano
-1 sprig fresh rosemary
-1 sprig fresh thyme
-1 tablespoon black peppercorns
-2 bay leaves
-½ tablespoon allspice berries
-½ tablespoon cloves
-Raw apple cider vinegar
-Raw honey to taste

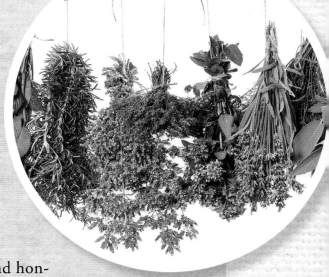

Place all ingredients (except vinegar and honey) in a quart glass jar. Cover with enough vinegar to cover contents by about two inches. Cover with a tight-fitting (non-metal) lid. Place jar in cupboard for at least four weeks (preferably longer). Shake the mixture once a day to help the maceration process. When ready, strain the liquid through a cheesecloth into a large mixing container. Add honey and stir thoroughly. Store the liquid in a glass bottle with a tight-fitting (non-metal) lid. Keep the bottle in a dark cupboard.

Spring Cleaning Oxymel

This oxymel targets residual malaise and gets the body going in the springtime. Rosehips and orange peel bring some tart and fruity zing to the composition. If fresh calendula flowers are available, increase their amount to a cup. You could also throw a handful of chopped fresh stinging nettle or dandelion leaves into this recipe.

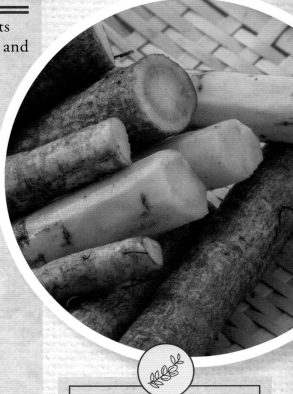

- –¾ cup fresh grated burdock root
- –½ cup dried calendula flowers
- –½ cup dried rose hips
- –½ cup peeled and sliced ginger
- –1 tablespoon dried orange peel
- –1 tablespoon fresh grated turmeric root
- –Raw apple cider vinegar
- –Raw honey to taste

Place all ingredients (except vinegar and honey) in a quart glass jar. Cover with enough vinegar to cover contents by about two inches. Cover with a tight-fitting (non-metal) lid. Place jar in cupboard for at least four weeks (preferably longer). Shake the mixture once a day to help the maceration process. When ready, strain the liquid through a cheesecloth into a large mixing container. Add honey and stir thoroughly. Store the liquid in a glass bottle with a tight-fitting (non-metal) lid. Keep the bottle in a dark cupboard.

After a long winter, burdock root is a helpful spring ally. It detoxifies the body, cleanses the blood, strengthens the lymphatic system, and inhibits the growth of bacteria in the body.

DIFFUSION

Diffusers are small electrical units that release water-based essential oil vapor into a room. Because they are unheated, the volatile compounds in the oils remain intact. Nebulizers also pump essential oil vapor into the air, but do it without water. Generally, you place a few drops of essential oil in a hand-blown glass container and turn on a small compressor that's connected with a piece of tubing. The glass unit disperses a fine mist of micro-particles mixed with the stream of air produced by the pump. This method increases the surface area of the oil molecules. It's an extremely effective way to disinfect and energize the atmosphere. Diffusers and nebulizers can be used in a sick room for 10 to 15 minutes every hour to clear airborne microbes that may spread infection.

Ceramic or metal rings designed to be placed directly on light bulbs are available online and at many stores. Place 2–3 drops on the ring while it's cold, and be sure not to touch it again until it cools down after turning off the light. You can also place a couple drops of essential oil directly on the bulb, although the oil doesn't last as long.

Clay and terra cotta discs and holders are the simplest of all. Add a few drops of oil to the disc surface and allow natural sunlight to heat up the surface and disperse the scent.

Spring Flowers Diffusion Blend

—**3 drops Roman chamomile oil**
—**3 drops lavender oil**
—**2 drops geranium oil**

Combine all oils and add to a diffuser.

With its floral notes and uplifting scent, this is the perfect blend to use when the weather warms up. But you don't have to wait: use it whenever you need some springtime in your life!

A Walk in the Woods Diffusion Blend

–4 drops frankincense oil
–3 drops fir oil
–3 drops pine oil
–2 drops cedarwood oil

Combine all oils and add to a diffuser.

This warm, woody blend promotes feelings of calm and relaxation. Try it in your home or office after a stressful day: the combination of clean, outdoorsy scents will transport you to the peacefulness of nature.

Chai Tea Diffusion Blend

–3 drops cardamom oil
–2 drops cassia oil
–2 drops clove oil
–1 drop black pepper oil
–1 drop ginger oil

Combine all oils and add to a diffuser.

Caution: this blend smells good enough to drink! With the spicy aroma of chai tea, this is a great blend to use in the kitchen. But it doesn't just smell good: the oils in this mix are known for their ability to calm nausea and lower blood pressure.

Pay Attention Diffusion Blend

–2 drops grapefruit oil
–2 drops lavender oil
–2 drops lemon oil
–2 drops peppermint oil
–1 drop basil oil
–1 drop rosemary oil

Combine all oils and add to a diffuser.

Having trouble focusing? The oils in this blend help you stay alert, while also decreasing your stress and anxiety. A great blend for students to use when preparing for an important exam. Or try it at the office when you need to complete a big project.

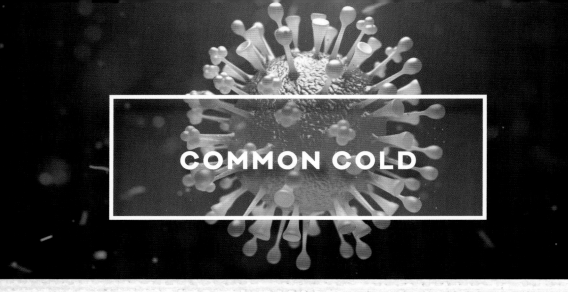

COMMON COLD

Every year Americans will suffer through more than one billion colds. That's one billion runny noses, coughs, sneezes, aches, and sore throats. Colds make such frequent appearances that the infection has come to be known as the "common cold."

Where's the Cold Vaccine?

Good question! One of the main reasons we don't yet have a vaccine for the cold is that viruses are just too hard to pin down. Viruses live inside cells, which means they are protected from most medicines in the bloodstream. So even if you took an antiviral drug, chances are your body wouldn't allow it to penetrate the cells. Another reason viruses are so difficult to kill is that they don't grow well in a laboratory setting. Their ultimate playground is an environment just like the inside of your nose.

Kitchen Cupboard Cures

Too sick to even go outside and get supplies during your unwanted downtime? If you have any of these in your cupboard, you're in luck.

Chicken soup. Science backs up what grandmothers knew all along—chicken soup does help a cold. Scientists believe it's the fumes in the soup that release the mucus in your nose and help your body better fight against its viral invaders. Chicken soup also contains cysteines, which are good at thinning mucus. And the soup provides easily absorbed nutrients.

Honey. Make your own cough syrup by mixing together ¼ cup honey and ¼ cup apple cider vinegar. Pour the mixture into a jar or bottle and seal tightly. Shake well before using. Take 1 tablespoon every four hours.

Hot peppers. Hot and spicy foods are notorious for making your nose run and your eyes water. The hot stuff in peppers is called capsaicin and is pharmacologically similar to guaifenesin, an expectorant found in some over-the-counter cough syrups. This similarity leads some experts to believe that eating hot foods can clear up mucus and ease stuffy noses.

Tea. A cup of hot tea with honey does the same trick as chicken soup; it loosens up your nasal passages and makes that stuffy nose feel better. Folk healers have known this secret for centuries. They often suggest drinking tea with spices and herbs that contain aromatic oils with antiviral properties. Try tea with elder, ginger, yarrow, mint, thyme, bee balm, lemon balm, catnip, garlic, onions, or mustard.

Yogurt. One study found that participants who ate ¾ cup yogurt a day before and during cold season had 25 percent fewer colds. But you've got to start early and maintain your yogurt eating throughout the peak cold season.

Vitamin Supplements

Vitamin C. It won't prevent a cold, but research shows that vitamin C can help reduce the length and severity of symptoms. But to reap the benefits, you've got to take a lot of it. The RDA for men and women 15 and older is 60 mg, but studies show that you'd need to take upward of 1,000 mg to 3,000 mg to get the cold-symptom-sparing rewards of vitamin C. For the short term, experts believe that wouldn't be harmful, but taking too much vitamin C for too long can cause severe diarrhea. Before loading up on vitamin C, check with your doctor.

Zinc. Studies have found that zinc may help immune cells fight a cold and may ease cold symptoms. The most effective zinc lozenges are those that contain 15 to 25 mg of zinc gluconate or zinc gluconate-glycine per lozenge. You can get the most out of your zinc lozenges if you start using them at the first sign of a cold and continue taking them for several days.

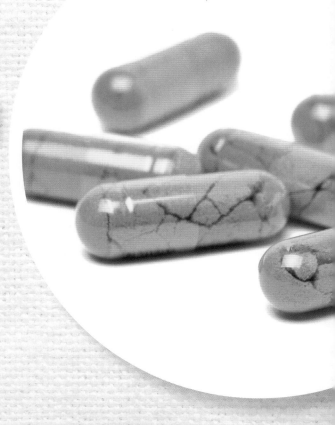

A Little Under the Weather Tea

This tea is good for when you feel a cold coming on or are already suffering a mild bout of respiratory illness. It's a warming tea that also helps clear congestion in the lungs.

- –3 tablespoons fennel seeds
- –3 tablespoons dried ginger pieces
- –3 tablespoons peppermint
- –2 tablespoons hyssop
- –1 tablespoon elecampane root
- –1 tablespoon cloves

Mix all ingredients thoroughly. When making tea, pour 1½ cups boiling water over 1 heaping tablespoon of mix. Steep for 10 minutes and strain. Add honey to taste.

Tea for Lingering Colds

Sometimes a cold or the remnant congestion just never seems to end. This mix addresses the lungs, sinuses, and throat, and is deeply refreshing.

- –2 tablespoons green tea
- –2 tablespoons dried elderberries
- –1 tablespoon echinacea
- –1 tablespoon elecampane root
- –1 tablespoon lemon balm
- –1 tablespoon rosemary
- –1 tablespoon slippery elm
- –1 tablespoon spearmint
- –1 tablespoon yarrow

Mix all ingredients thoroughly. When making tea, pour 1½ cups boiling water over 1 heaping tablespoon of mix. Steep for 10 minutes and strain. Add honey to taste.

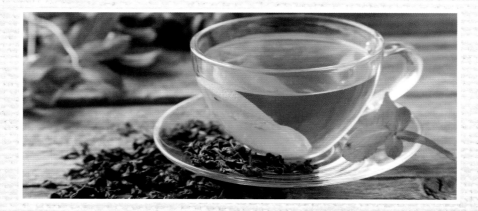

Breathe Easy Diffusion Blend

- 2 drops eucalyptus oil
- 2 drops lemon oil
- 2 drops peppermint oil
- 1 drop clove oil
- 1 drop lime oil
- 1 drop rosemary oil

This blend is perfect to use during cold and flu season. The oils work together to protect against infection, support respiratory function, and clear up congestion.

Immunity-Boosting Diffusion Blend

- 3 drops clove oil
- 3 drops lemon oil
- 2 drops cinnamon oil
- 2 drops eucalyptus oil
- 1 drop rosemary oil

This blend seems to fill a room with brisk and sparkling good cheer. Every oil is a powerhouse antimicrobial.

Cold Remedy Diffusion Blend

- 5 drops rosemary oil
- 4 drops eucalyptus oil
- 4 drops peppermint oil
- 3 drops cypress oil
- 2 drops lemon oil

If you prefer to try natural remedies before perusing the pharmacy's cold medicine aisle, this blend is for you. Rosemary calms aches and pains and relieves nausea, while eucalyptus and peppermint ease congestion. Cypress helps quell coughs, and a bit of lemon fights fatigue. Everything you need in a cold remedy in one blend!

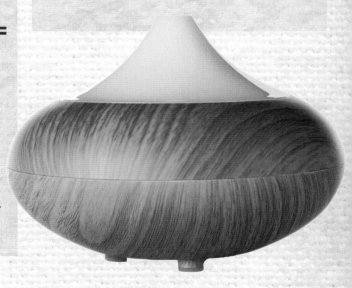

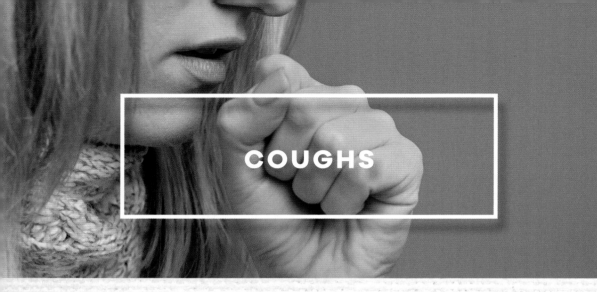

COUGHS

Annoying and disruptive, a persistent cough can put a damper on your daily routine. Coughs can be defined by how long they last. A brief cough is caused by such factors as cold air, irritating fumes, breathing dust, or drawing food into the airways. A persistent cough, however, typically results from mucus and other secretions brought on by respiratory disorders such as the cold, the flu, pneumonia, or tuberculosis. Some remedies aim to moisten dry throats, while others are expectorants, helping you cough up and get rid of mucus and irritants.

Kitchen Cupboard Cures

Garlic. It's full of antibiotic and antiviral properties, plus garlic is also an expectorant, so it helps you cough up stubborn bacteria and/or mucus that are languishing in your lungs. Some experts advise that to reap garlic's full cold- and flu-fighting benefits, you have to eat it raw. Yet swallowing 4 to 8 raw garlic cloves a day (the recommended amount) is hard for most people to stomach. Cheat a little by mixing the cloves into plain yogurt and putting a dollop on your soup. A cup of garlic broth may do the trick for your cough, too, and it is easy to prepare. Smash 1 to 3 cloves garlic, add 2 quarts water, and cook on low heat for one hour.

Honey. Honey has long been used in traditional Chinese medicine for coughs because it's a natural expectorant, promoting the flow of mucus. This is the simple recipe: Mix 1 tablespoon honey into 1 cup hot water and enjoy. Now how sweet is that? Squeeze some lemon juice in if you want a little tartness. Before bedtime, adults may add 1 tablespoon brandy or whiskey to aid in sleep.

Pepper. Pepper is a bit of an irritant, but this characteristic is a plus for those suffering from coughs accompanied by thick mucus. The irritating property of pepper stimulates circulation and the flow of mucus in the airways and sinuses. Place 1 teaspoon black pepper into a cup and sweeten things up with the addition of 1 tablespoon honey. Fill with boiling water, steep for 10 to 15 minutes, stir, and sip.

Thyme. Store-bought cough syrups are often so medicinal-tasting that it's hard to get them down. This version is guaranteed to go down the hatch easily. Thyme and peppermint help clear congested air passages and have antimicrobial and antispasmodic properties to relieve the hacking. Mullein and licorice soothe irritated membranes and help reduce inflammation. Combine 2 teaspoons each dried thyme, peppermint, mullein, and licorice root into 1 cup boiling water. Cover and steep for half an hour. Strain and add ½ cup honey. If the honey doesn't dissolve, heat the tea gently and stir. Store in the refrigerator in a covered container for up to three months. Take 1 teaspoon as needed.

Vapor Balm

A vapor balm (a salve containing essential oils) or massage oil can be rubbed over the chest, back, and throat to relieve congestion. Vapor balms increase circulation and warmth in the chest as they are absorbed through the skin. Placing a flannel cloth on the chest after rubbing in the oil will increase the warming action. Commercial products, such as Vicks VapoRub, still use derivatives of essential oils (or their synthetic oil counterparts) such as thymol from thyme and menthol from mint, in a petroleum ointment base, but more natural alternatives are available from your health store. Essential oil molecules are also easily inhaled from the balm.

Therapeutic Steam

To create a therapeutic steam, add a few drops of essential oil to a pan of water that is simmering on the stove. You can also use a humidifier—some actually provide a compartment for essential oils. If you are at the office or traveling and steaming is impractical, try inhaling a tissue scented with the oils, or use a natural nasal inhaler. These are available in health stores and are found online, or you can make your own. If you don't have a diffuser but would like to disinfect the air, simply combine water and essential oils and dispense the solution from a spray bottle.

Vapor Rub

- 12 drops eucalyptus oil
- 5 drops peppermint oil
- 5 drops thyme oil
- 1 ounce olive oil

Combine ingredients in a glass bottle. Shake well to mix oils evenly. Gently massage into chest and throat. Use one to five times per day and especially just before bed.

CUTS AND SCRAPES

Simple cuts and scrapes can easily be treated with antiseptic essential oils. A mist of diluted oil is an excellent way to apply them. Herbal salves containing antiseptic essential oils are also effective in treating scrapes or wounds that aren't too deep. Need to protect your cut? Many of the resins and balsams such as benzoin, frankincense, and myrrh actually form a protective barrier over the wound that acts as an antiseptic "Band-Aid." In an emergency, don't forget that you can dab a little lavender or tea tree oil directly on a scrape.

Essential Oils for Cuts and Scrapes

- **Benzoin**
- **Eucalyptus**
- **Frankincense**
- **Geranium**
- **Lavender**
- **Lemon**
- **Myrrh**
- **Rose**
- **Tea tree**

Germ Fighter Spray

- –12 drops tea tree oil
- –6 drops eucalyptus oil
- –6 drops lemon oil
- –2 ounces distilled water

Combine the ingredients in a glass spray bottle and shake well to disperse the oils before each use. As an alternative to the distilled water, you can use a tincture made from an antiseptic herb such as Oregon grape root. If you do this, keep in mind that tinctures contain alcohol, which will make the essential oils disperse better and increase the antiseptic properties of the spray, but it will also sting more on an open wound. Apply immediately and then several times a day to keep the wound clean and encourage healing.

DENTAL DECAY

Our teeth serve us well when they're in good order, but when something goes wrong, ouch! First comes that off-and-on-again little twinge, the one we ignore and hope will disappear. Next comes the sensitivity to hot and cold. And finally, the full-out throb that hurts so bad that pulling the tooth out with a piece of string tied to a doorknob doesn't seem like such a bad way out. Serious dental problems require the attention of a dentist. But minor gum ailments and toothaches can be alleviated, at least temporarily, with the following remedies.

Kitchen Cupboard Cures

Allspice. It helps relieve toothache. Wet your finger and dip it into the ground spice, then rub it along the gum line near the aching tooth. You can also steep some in a glass of warm water, then rinse your mouth with it. Not only does this rinse relieve pain, it also freshens your breath.

Cheese. You know those nasty bacteria that are just waiting to take a whack at your tooth enamel? Cheese is their sworn enemy. First, it stimulates the salivary glands to clean the mouth. According to studies, just a few ounces of hard cheese eaten after a meal may protect against decay. There's also evidence to suggest that fatty acids in cheese may have antibacterial properties. And finally, cheese proteins may actually coat and protect tooth enamel.

Cloves. Cloves contain eugenol, a chemical with natural antiseptic and anesthetic properties. That explains why ground cloves have been used to relieve toothaches for thousands of years. Moisten 1 teaspoon powdered cloves in olive oil and pack it against an aching cavity. Dentists still use a mixture of eugenol and zinc oxide before applying amalgam when filling teeth.

Coriander. This spice, as well as thyme and green tea, has antibacterial properties. Brew a tea from your choice of the three and use as a mouth rinse after meals.

Sage. Add 2 teaspoons sage to 2 cups water, then boil. Cool for 15 minutes, then swish in your mouth for several minutes. Sage has an antibacterial property that may reduce decay.

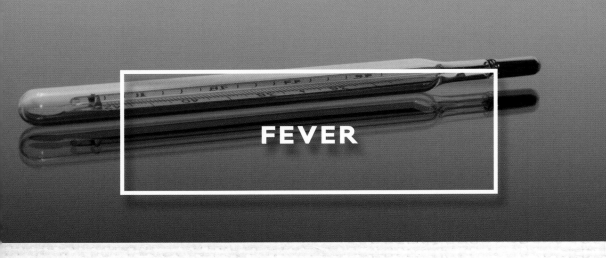

FEVER

Fever is a good thing. It's your body's attempt to kill off invading bacteria and other nasty organisms that can't survive the heat. The hypothalamus, which is the body's thermostat, senses the assault on the body and turns up the heat much the way you turn up the thermostat when you feel cold. It's a simple defense mechanism, and the sweat that comes with a fever is merely a way to cool the body down.

Kitchen Cupboard Cures

Basil. Mix 1 teaspoon basil with ¼ teaspoon black pepper. Steep in 1 cup hot water to make a tea. Add 1 teaspoon honey. Drink two to three times a day.

Blackberry vinegar. This is a great fever elixir, but it takes several days to prepare. Pour cider vinegar over a pound or two of blackberries, then cover the container and store it in a cool, dark place for three days. Strain for a day, since it takes time for all the liquid to drain from the berries, and collect the liquid in another container. Then add 2 cups sugar to each 2½ cups juice. Bring to a boil, then simmer for 5 minutes while you skim the scum off the top. Cool and store in an airtight jar in a cool place. Mix 1 teaspoonful with water to quench the thirst caused by a fever.

Cilantro. Nice, fresh cilantro can be turned into a simple fever remedy. Wash thoroughly and place a handful of leaves in a blender with ⅓ cup water. Blend thoroughly, then strain, reserving the liquid. Take 2 teaspoons of the liquid three times a day.

Ginger. This can help break a high fever. Grate 2 tablespoons fresh ginger and add to 2 cups boiling water. Steep 30 minutes. Add a little honey to sweeten, and drink a cup of the warm beverage every two to three hours.

Oregano and marjoram. A tea made from a mixture of some spice rack staples can help reduce fever. Steep 1 teaspoon each of oregano and marjoram in a pint of boiling water for 30 minutes. Strain, and drink warm a couple times a day. Refrigerate unused portion until needed, then gently warm.

Pineapple. Fresh is best. It's one of nature's anti-inflammatory agents that can fight fever. Pineapple is also packed with juice that can prevent dehydration.

Sage. Mix 2 teaspoons dried sage with 1 teaspoon dried peppermint. Pour 1 cup boiling water over these and steep 15 minutes. Strain and sweeten with honey. Drink 2 to 3 cups per day, rewarmed. Add a little honey to sweeten the taste.

Herbs That Will Make You Sweat

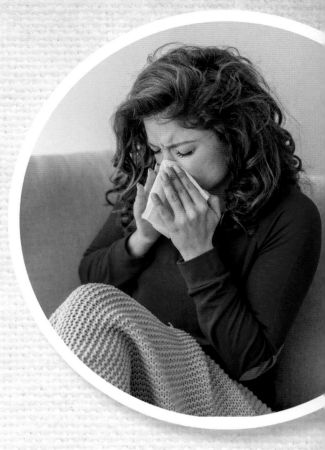

Many traditional folk fever remedies are called diaphoretics, meaning they'll make you sweat. Properties in the following diaphoretic herbs increase blood circulation to the skin, which brings on the sweat. And that's a good thing because sweating cools the body during a fever. Take any of the following herbs as hot teas: agueweed, boneset, bupleurum, catnip, dandelion root and leaves, elderberries and flowers, feverfew, ginseng, strawberry leaf, and yarrow. Just be sure to drink plenty of water, because sweating can cause dehydration. Then go to bed and get some rest.

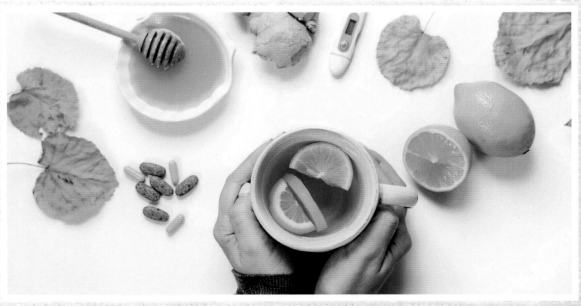

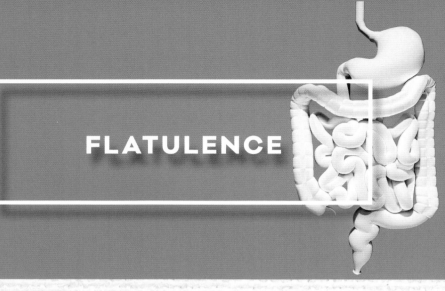

FLATULENCE

Gas happens. Called flatus, or flatulence when it finally does escape, it's normal. Its beginnings are in the foods we eat. We eat, therefore we pass gas. Our stomach acids are breaking down last night's pasta primavera into elements that will either be absorbed into the body or eliminated. And that breakdown causes gas.

Bodily gas originates in the stomach and travels down to the intestines (unless it comes back up as a belch). Its construction is pretty simple: carbon dioxide, hydrogen, nitrogen, and methane. Well, those gases make up about 99 percent of the gas we pass. The other 1 percent is divided among up to 250 different gases, all of which occur naturally when carbohydrates are broken down. If you swallow air, you add oxygen to the mix.

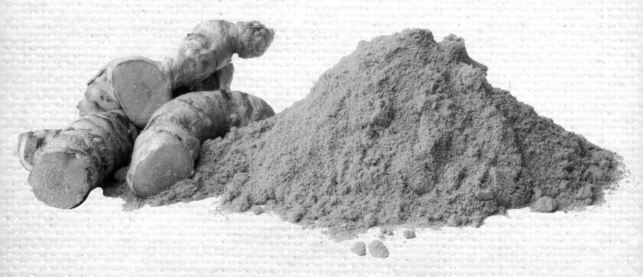

Kitchen Cupboard Cures

Caraway. Caraway seeds and their oils are carminatives (they get rid of gas), but who wants to eat just the seeds? Caraway seed crackers and breads with caraway seeds are a tasty way to make your system gas-unfriendly. Caraway may also be more palatable in a tea.

Cloves. They pep up digestion and eliminate gas. Add 2 to 3 whole cloves to rice before cooking. Sprinkle on apples and pears when baking. Or steep 2 to 3 whole cloves in a cup of boiling water for ten minutes, sweeten to taste, and drink.

Coriander. This helps in the downward movement of foods being digested and can ease cramps, hiccups, bloating, and flatulence. Crush the seeds into powder and add to foods such as vegetable stir-fry. Its flavor really enhances curry and Middle Eastern dishes, too.

Fennel seeds. It's an acquired taste, but it may be one well worth acquiring if you're plagued by gas. Fennel's digestive powers are so good that in India fennel is customarily eaten after a meal to help digestion and freshen the breath.

For gas, drink it as a tea by steeping ½ teaspoon seeds in 1 cup boiling water for ten minutes. Or, sprinkle them over those gassy vegetables during cooking or add to stir-fries. If you've acquired the taste, fennel also works well cooked into figs, apples, pears, and plums.

Rosemary. If you're eating a gassy food, sprinkle on a little rosemary to cut down the effect. You can do the same with sage and thyme, too.

Turmeric. This may stop a gas problem altogether. Turmeric is one of the many flavorful and curative spices found in curry powder. You can add turmeric itself to rice or season a bland dish with curry powder, which contains turmeric. However you use it, it helps alleviate gas.

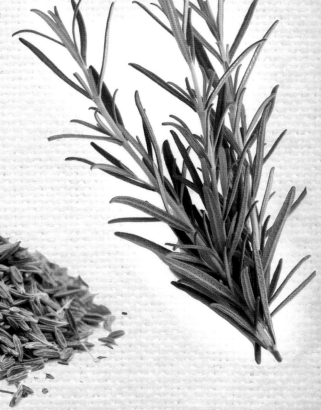

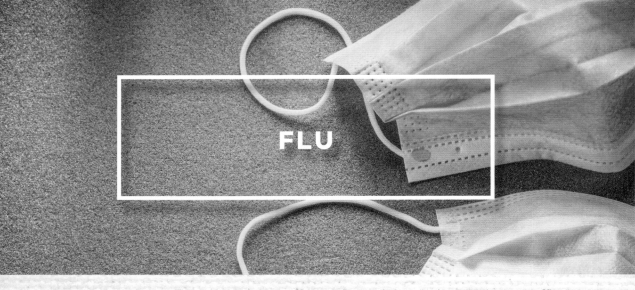

FLU

Unlike the common cold, which causes a stuffy nose, sore throat, and sneezing, the flu is a viral infection that strikes the entire body with a vengeance. The misery starts suddenly with chills and fever and spirals into more unpleasant symptoms that will take you out of commission: a sore throat, dry cough, stuffy or runny nose, headache, nausea, vomiting, severe muscle aches and pains, weakness, backache, and loss of appetite. Some people even experience pain and stiffness in the joints.

Kitchen Cupboard Cures

Honey. A hacking cough can keep you and every other household member up all night. Keep the peace with honey. Honey has long been used in traditional medicine for coughs. It's a simple enough recipe: Mix 1 tablespoon honey into 1 cup hot water, stir well, and enjoy. Honey acts as a natural expectorant, promoting the flow of mucus. Squeeze some lemon in if you want a little tartness.

Pepper. Pepper is an irritant (try sniffling some), yet this annoying characteristic is a plus for those suffering from coughs with thick mucus. The irritating property of pepper stimulates circulation and the flow of mucus. Place 1 teaspoon black pepper into a cup and sweeten things up with the addition of 1 tablespoon honey. Fill with boiling water, let steep for 10 to 15 minutes, stir, and sip.

Tea. A cup of hot tea is just another way to take your fluids, which are so essential when you have the flu. Just be sure to choose decaffeinated varieties. Caffeine is a mild diuretic, which is counterproductive when you have the flu, and you certainly don't want to be awakened with the need to use the bathroom when you need your rest!

Thyme. It's time to try thyme when the mucous membranes are stuffed, the head aches, and the body is hot with fever. Wonderfully fragrant, thyme delights the senses (if you can smell when sick) and works as a powerful expectorant and antiseptic, thanks to its constituent oil, thymol. By cupping your hands around a mug of thyme tea and breathing in the steam, the thymol sets to work through your upper respiratory tract, loosening mucus and inhibiting bacteria from settling down to stay. Make thyme tea in a snap by adding 1 teaspoon dried thyme leaves to 1 cup boiling water. Let steep for five minutes while inhaling the steam. Strain the tea, sweeten with honey (to taste), and slowly sip.

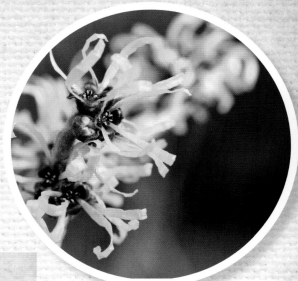

Germs-Be-Gone Spray

Surrounded by ailing relatives, coworkers, or friends all reeling from this year's most wicked flu strain? This spray will help you battle the bug.

- —8 drops cinnamon oil
- —8 drops clove oil
- —8 drops eucalyptus oil
- —8 drops lemon oil
- —8 drops rosemary oil
- —2 ounces witch hazel
- —8 ounces water

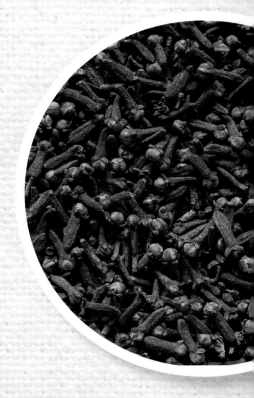

Fill a glass spray bottle with all ingredients. Shake well before use. Spray the air, tabletops, counters, doorknobs, and anywhere else you think the flu bug might be. it will also sting more on an open wound. Apply immediately and then several times a day to keep the wound clean and encourage healing.

Herbs to the Rescue

Peppermint tea is an excellent ally to have on hand during flu season. Running a high fever is common with the flu. A way to cool your hot head, via sweating, is with a cup of peppermint tea. As an added bonus, peppermint contains menthol, which works as a decongestant to help unstuff sinuses. And peppermint has antispasmodic properties to help that hack.

A combination of thyme and peppermint makes an effective steam broth that will deliver healing aromas to your aching nose and throat. Combine 1½ quarts boiling water and 2 tablespoons each of dried thyme and peppermint in a large pot. Cover and steep for five minutes. Place the pot on a table and remove the lid. Lean in and cover both your head and the pot of steaming herbs with a large towel. Slowly breathe the herbal broth for 15 minutes.

All of the plants in this book have healing properties, and most of them have compounds that will ease or heal the body during bouts of respiratory illnesses like colds and the flu. Besides honey, pepper, peppermint, tea, and thyme, here are some other standouts that are especially effective at alleviating or shortening the duration of the flu.

- **Cinnamon**
- **Bergamot**
- **Garlic**
- **Elderberry**
- **Oregano**
- **Propolis**
- **Ravensara**
- **Rosemary**
- **Sage**

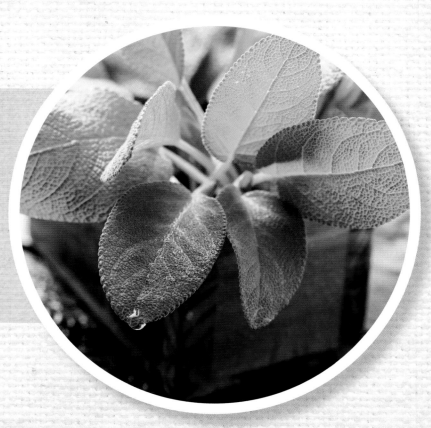

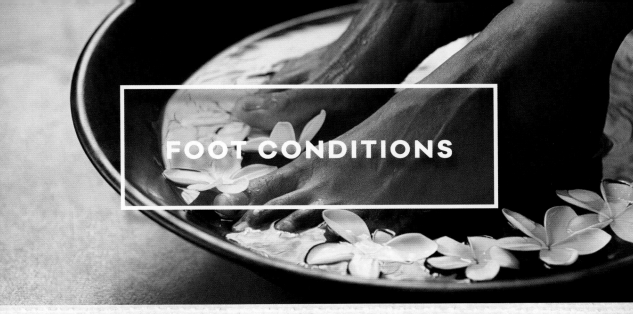

FOOT CONDITIONS

Pathogens associated with the feet are bacterial or fungal. In the case of excessive foot odor, known in the medical profession as bromhidrosis, the culprit may be bacteria. Some bacteria find your moist and warm feet, socks, and shoes the perfect place to breed and multiply. Thousands of sweat glands on the soles of the feet produce perspiration composed of water, sodium chloride, fat, minerals, and various acids that are the end products of your body's metabolism. In the presence of certain bacteria (namely those found in dark, damp shoes), these sweaty secretions break down, generating the stench that turns people green. Certain fungi are also attracted to the moist environment found surrounding feet cloistered in socks and shoes. Most people are familiar with athlete's foot because it is so common. What they might not know is that it is a fungal infection. The perfect natural antibiotic solution to these foot problems is essential oils.

Treatments

If sweating feet are part of the problem, you can use sage to decrease perspiration. Peppermint will help relieve the itching that accompanies a fungal infection. Incorporating the essential oils into a cornstarch powder or a vinegar-based preparation will discourage fungal growth because both are quite drying. Vinegar has the extra benefit of destroying fungal infections.

Some of the most effective antifungal essential oils are tea tree and eucalyptus. Lavender, myrrh, and geranium are close seconds. A small amount of peppermint essential oil relieves the itching, and since it stimulates blood circulation, it helps perk you up after a long day on your feet. Don't hesitate to use the same essential oils to treat funguses that creep under nails or affect other parts of the body.

An aromatic foot bath is one great way to treat fungal conditions like athlete's foot or to simply revitalize feet after a long day. You simply can't ask for a better way to take your medicine! Get yourself a basin large enough to accommodate both feet comfortably, fill it with warm water, and add several drops of essential oil. Add Epsom salts to relax tight muscles and soreness.

For a complete anti-fungal treatment, start off with a foot bath, hand soak, or wash that covers the afflicted area. Afterward, dry off thoroughly, then apply the Fungal Fighter Solution with vinegar followed by the Fungal Fighter Powder. Do the entire routine at least once a day, and apply either the vinegar or the powder a few extra times.

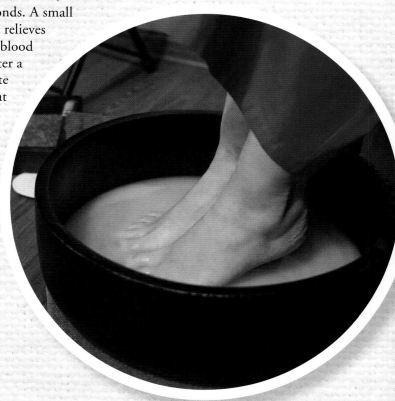

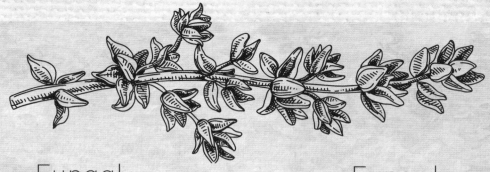

Fungal Fighter Solution

–12 drops tea tree oil

–8 drops geranium oil

–3 drops thyme oil

–2 drops myrrh oil

–1 tablespoon tincture of benzoin

–2 ounces apple cider vinegar

Combine ingredients in a small bottle (remember—no metal caps when using vinegar) and shake well before each use. Dab this solution on the afflicted or use it as a wash at least once a day—more if possible. Tincture of benzoin can be found online and at some drugstores.

Fungal Fighter Powder

–14 drops eucalyptus or tea tree oil

–8 drops geranium oil

–5 drops sage oil

–1 drop peppermint oil

–¼ cup cornstarch

Place the cornstarch in a resealable plastic bag. Sprinkle in the essential oils slowly, trying to distribute them evenly through the powder. Close the bag and toss the powder, breaking up any clumps that form. For long-term storage, keep the powder in a glass or ceramic container, although you probably will find a shake bottle with a perforated lid more convenient to dispense it. Use at least once a day, more often if possible.

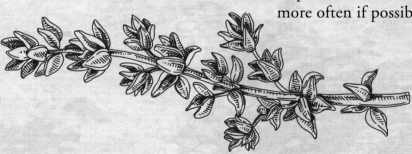

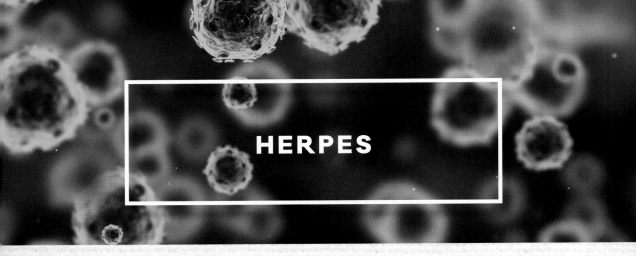

HERPES

Herpes is a painful viral infection that appears on the genitals or around the mouth in the form of fever blisters. The herpes virus can lay dormant in the nervous system for a long time. Current conventional medicine has little to offer to treat herpes and does not know how to completely eliminate the virus. The virus reactivates when the immune system is weakened, such as when you are under emotional or physical stress. Consider using aromatherapy and other methods to build up your immune system and to relax.

Research shows that creams made from capsaicin, a compound found in cayenne, will deaden the pain of herpes and shingles. The essential oils of cayenne will also work if added to a cream or oil base, but extremely careful with it since too much of this oil can burn the skin.

Tea tree and niaouli are two favorite essential oils to treat herpes. Myrrh essential oil is also very effective. Dilute the essential oil of your choice in an equal amount of carrier oil or alcohol, and apply it directly to the herpes blisters. If applied as soon as the blisters begin to appear, any of these oils may prevent it from breaking out. This formula can be used on another virus related to herpes, called herpes zoster, which causes chicken pox and shingles.

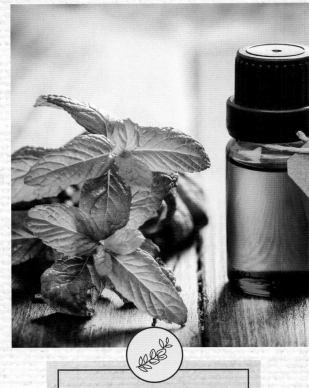

Small amounts of peppermint oil sometimes diminish the nerve-tingling pain of herpes and shingles.

Herpes Relief Formula 1

- 10 drops tea tree oil
- 5 drops myrrh oil
- 5 drops geranium or bergamot oil
- 2 drops peppermint oil
- ½ ounce carrier oil

Combine the ingredients and shake or stir well. Apply directly to affected area three to five times a day during an outbreak. If you would prefer a less oily formula, you can substitute either rubbing alcohol or vodka for the carrier oil, but try a little first to make sure the alcohol doesn't sting too much.

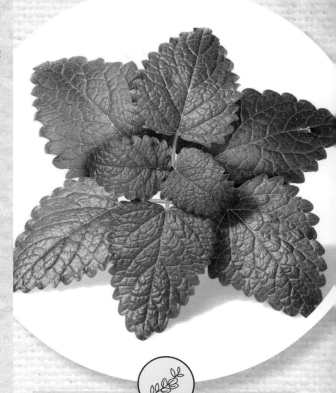

Herpes Relief Formula 2

- 8 drops tea tree oil
- 6 drops geranium oil
- 6 drops German chamomile oil
- 6 drops lavender oil
- 3 drops lemon oil

Combine ingredients and put one drop of mixture on a moist cotton ball. Dab gently over affected area.

Lemon balm, or Melissa (*Melissa officinalis*) essential oil has excellent antiviral properties that make it a useful treatment for some herpes sufferers. The oil is applied neat, directly to the location of the outbreak. This remedy may be too irritating for the skin of some users, however. If you try this treatment, first dilute it with a carrier oil.

SORE THROAT

It's scratchy, tender, and swollen, and you dread the simple task of swallowing. But you must swallow, and when you do, you brace yourself for the unavoidable pain. The mechanics of a sore throat are pretty simple. It's an inflammation of the pharynx, which is the tube that extends from the back of the mouth to the esophagus. A sore throat may be caused by a viral infection (colds, flu, etc.) or a bacterial infection (strep throat, for example). It may also arise from smoking, acid reflux, allergies, throat abuse from singing or shouting, or infected tonsils. Whatever the cause, you want a quick cure when your throat is on fire.

Kitchen Cupboard Cures

Cinnamon. Mix 2 parts cinnamon, 2 parts ginger, and 3 parts licorice powder. Steep 1 teaspoon of this mixture in 1 cup boiling water for ten minutes, then drink as a sore throat cure three times a day.

Garlic. This Amish remedy can treat or prevent sore throats. Peel a fresh clove, slice it in half, and place 1 piece in each cheek. Suck on the garlic like a cough drop. Occasionally, crush your teeth against the garlic, not to bite it in half, but to release its allicin, a chemical that can kill the bacteria that causes strep. Onions may be used as well, as they also contain allicin.

Horseradish. Try this Russian sore throat cure. Combine 1 tablespoon pure horseradish or horseradish root with 1 teaspoon honey and 1 teaspoon ground cloves. Mix in a glass of warm water and drink slowly.

Marjoram. Make a soothing tea with a spoonful of marjoram steeped in a cup of boiling water for ten minutes. Strain, then sweeten to taste with honey.

Sage. This curative herb is a great sore throat gargle. Mix 1 teaspoon in 1 cup boiling water. Steep for ten minutes, then strain. Add 1 teaspoon each cider vinegar and honey, then gargle four times a day.

Turmeric. Try this gargle to calm a cranky throat, or try the turmeric-touting recipe on the next page. Mix together 1 cup hot water, ½ teaspoon turmeric, and ½ teaspoon salt. Gargle with the mixture twice a day. If you're not good with the gargle, mix ½ teaspoon turmeric in 1 cup hot milk and drink.

Bulletproof Golden Milk

This take on traditional golden milk features extra spices to bolster your body's defenses. It's delicious and goes down smoothly. You can substitute the coconut milk with regular milk.

- 2 cups coconut milk
- 1 teaspoon coconut oil or ghee
- 1 teaspoon ground turmeric
- ¾ teaspoon grated fresh ginger
- ¼ teaspoon ground cinnamon
- ¼ teaspoon ground cardamom
- Freshly crushed black pepper to taste
- 1 dash ground clove
- Honey to taste

Heat all ingredients except honey in pot and simmer covered for 10 to 15 minutes. Strain and stir in honey.

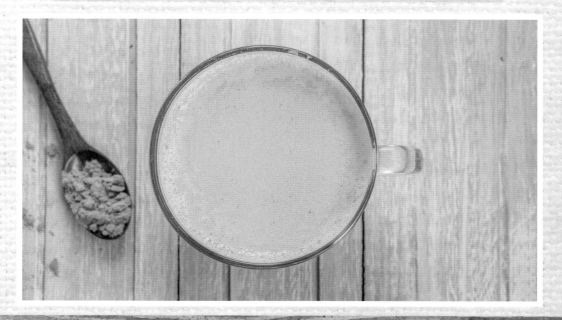

Essential Oils

Herbal teas of sage, hyssop, and thyme are good gargles for a sore throat. The essential oils of these plants can be diluted as well. This brings the antibacterial and soothing essential oils into direct contact with the bacteria responsible for causing a sore throat or laryngitis. In an emergency, a few drops of essential oil diluted in two ounces of water may also be used. Other essential oils good for a sore throat include bergamot, eucalyptus, lavender, lemon, sandalwood, tea tree, and thyme.

Neck Wrap

A simple neck wrap can ease discomfort. Mix a few drops of bergamot, lavender, and tea tree in a cup of hot water and soak a soft cloth (preferably flannel) in the water and wring it out. Wrap it around the neck. Cover with a towel to hold in the heat.

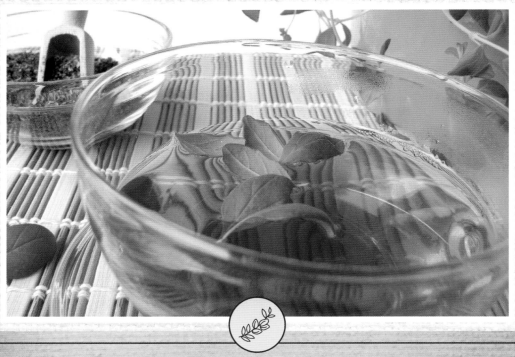

For centuries, European singers have known the secret to preserving their voices with aromatherapy and herbal remedies. Their most popular sore throat and laryngitis cure has been to gargle with a marjoram herb tea that has been sweetened with honey. You can also use the essential oil of marjoram to make a similar remedy. As both an antiseptic and anti-inflammatory, marjoram is a good choice.

URINARY TRACT INFECTIONS

Urinary tract infections (UTIs) are the second most common reason people visit their doctors each year. Men get UTIs, but they are much more common in women. If you've ever had a UTI, you'll probably never forget the symptoms. It usually starts with a sudden and frequent need to visit the bathroom. When you get there, you can squeeze out only a little bit of urine, and that's usually accompanied by a burning sensation in your bladder and/or urethra. In more extreme cases you may end up with fever, chills, back pain, and even blood in your urine. UTIs that last longer than two days require medical intervention. Untreated UTIs can infect the kidneys and turn into a much more serious problem. To help prevent a UTI from developing or nip one in the bud, try some of the remedies available in your own kitchen.

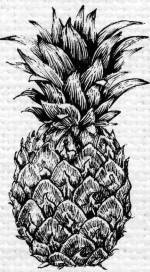

Kitchen Cupboard Cures

Blueberries. Blueberries and cranberries are from the same plant family and seem to have the same bacteria-inhibiting properties. In one study, blueberry juice was found to prevent UTIs. Although uncommon, it can be found in health food stores and some grocery stores.

Cranberry juice. Many studies have found that drinking cranberry juice may help you avoid urinary tract infections. It appears that cranberry juice prevents infection-causing bacteria from bedding down in your bladder, and it also has a very mild antibiotic effect. Drinking as little as 4 ounces of cranberry juice a day can help keep your bladder infection-free.

Pineapple. Bromelain is an enzyme found in pineapples. In one study, people with a UTI who were given bromelain along with their usual round of antibiotics got rid of their infection. Only half the people who were given a placebo plus an antibiotic showed no signs of lingering infection.

Essential Oils

Bergamot, cedarwood, chamomile, cypress, fir, frankincense, juniper berry, pine, sandalwood, tea tree, and bergamot are all especially effective oils for UTIs. However, juniper berry is so strong that it could irritate the kidneys if the bladder infection has spread into them. If that is the case, stick to the other oils. In fact, if there is any chance that you have a kidney infection, be sure to seek a doctor's opinion, as it can have serious consequences.

Bladder Infection Oil

- **8 drops juniper berry or cypress oil**
- **6 drops tea tree oil**
- **6 drops bergamot oil**
- **2 drops fennel oil**
- **2 ounces carrier oil**

Apply a massage oil or a compress containing the essential oils over the bladder, which is located under the lower abdomen, once or twice daily as an adjunct to herbal, nutritional, or even drug treatments. Added to a bath, these same essential oils can be used during an active infection and will help prevent future infections. If taking a full bath isn't practical, then try a sitz bath.

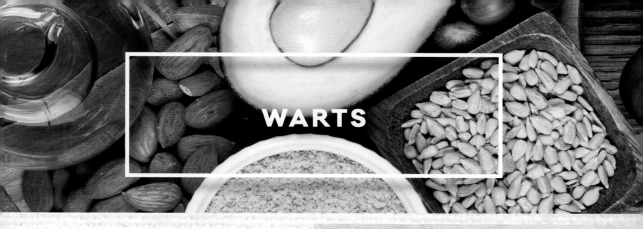

WARTS

Warts are raised areas on the skin that are often bumpy and dark in color. Genital warts are caused by the human papilloma virus (HPV). Difficult to detect, genital warts will temporarily turn whitish if you dab on vinegar that has been diluted in an equal amount of water.

Tea tree and particularly thuja essential oils are two of the most effective wart removers. Thuja is very strong, so use it carefully. Essential oils often get rid of warts, although the virus does stay in the system and can pop out again. Efficacy of treatment seems to depend on the individual—sometimes essential oils are effective and sometimes they aren't.

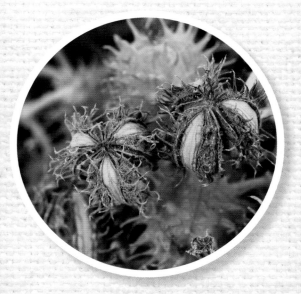

Wart Be Gone Oil

–12 drops tea tree oil
–12 drops thuja oil
–1 teaspoon castor oil
–800 IU vitamin E oil

Combine the ingredients. Apply directly to the wart(s) two to four times daily. Castor oil is a good choice of oil since it is a folk treatment for warts. This is a high concentration of essential oil, and thuja is particularly strong, so use a glass rod applicator, dropper, or cotton swab to apply and be sure not to get it on the skin around the wart since repeated use can burn sensitive skin.

Castor oil comes from the castor bean. The beans are poisonous but the extracted oil can be used topically. Traditionally, it has been used for skin conditions and to enhance skin health.

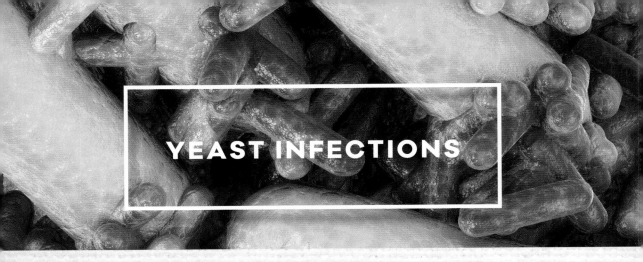

YEAST INFECTIONS

A yeast infection is a fungus that can proliferate anywhere the breeding ground is right. And the breeding ground is right in the genital and oral areas because that's where *Candida albicans*, the fungus that causes a yeast infection, lives. Yeast happens when the acidity of normal fluids is altered. Usually they're acidic enough to keep the yeast from flourishing. But when something goes wrong, the balance is tipped and the yeast have a party, multiplying over and over.

Typical yeast infections can be cured with remedies found on the pharmacy shelf either in cream or suppository form. There are also prescription medications available that will stop the problem in as little as three days. But if these are not available, there are also simple kitchen panaceas that can bring relief or cure and even stop the disease from recurring.

Basil. For thrush, make a basil tea and use it as a gargle. Boil 3½ cups water, remove from heat, and add 1¼ teaspoons ground basil. Cover and steep for 30 minutes. Cool and gargle. Or sweeten to taste with maple syrup and drink 1 cup twice a day.

Cranberry juice. Drunk unsweetened, it may acidify vaginal secretions and equip them to fight off the yeast.

Garlic. Eating 2 fresh garlic cloves a day, either plain or minced and tossed in a salad or sauce, may prevent yeast infections or help clear up a case of thrush.

Rosemary. To relieve itching and burning, make a tea of rosemary, and use it as a douche or dab it onto the external area.

Thyme. Make a thyme tea using 1 teaspoon dried thyme per 1 cup boiling water. Steep and drink 1 to 4 cups per day if you have a yeast infection.

Yogurt. The live culture in plain yogurt is a great remedy for a yeast infection, helping to restore the acid-bacteria balance in more ways than one.

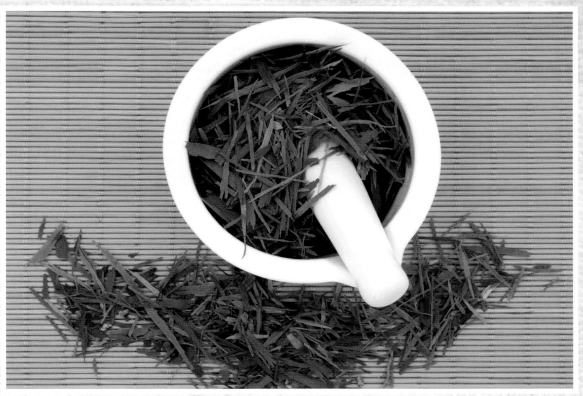

Indigenous peoples of the Amazon basin have used pau d'arco for centuries as a remedy for a variety of ailments, including malaria, respiratory illnesses, fever, arthritis, and fungal infections. It is especially effective against yeast infections.

Candida Fighter Tea

- –5 tablespoons pau d'arco
- –2 tablespoons thyme
- –1 tablespoon mint
- –1 tablespoon calendula
- –½ tablespoon oregano
- –½ tablespoon cloves

Mix all ingredients and store in a tea container. When ready to use, pour one cup boiling water over one tablespoon of tea mix. Steep for 10 minutes and strain.

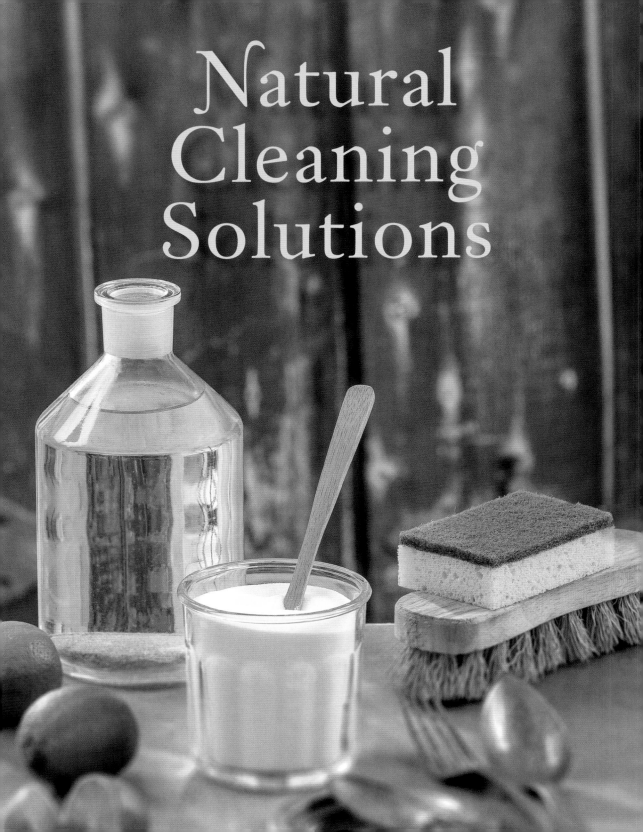

Natural
Cleaning
Solutions

The sheer variety of powerful, specialized chemical cleaners that consumers have access to in the marketplace is, on one hand, an example of the spectacular accomplishments of modern chemistry. On the other hand, it offers us the vista of slowly growing environmental degradation—toxins in our soils, polluted air and drinking water, and decreasing biodiversity.

Enter natural essential oils. Most are environmentally friendly and can take the place of dangerous cleaning chemicals. With a little knowledge, essential oils can be substituted for chemical cleaners. They can be used to kill bathroom mold, disinfect countertops, and repel pests and vermin. And they can do these things without leaving residual toxins that make their way into our bodies and down our drains.

There's another reason for using essential oils for housecleaning—they smell fantastic! Some people are very sensitive to the harsh and powerful fumes of commercial cleaners. They find it necessary to open windows and doors while cleaning and stay out of the rooms they've cleaned until the smells have dissipated. This is hardly the case with essential oils. In fact, cleaning with essential oils can be a pleasure. The sparkling clean scents of pine, lemon, lime, and tea tree are naturally uplifting. Lingering aromas like cedar, lavender, clary sage, and basil reinforce the feeling of a job well done.

Making your own essential-oil-based cleaning recipes doesn't take much time. It isn't expensive either. But you will want to use dark-tinted cleaning containers and spray bottles that are made of glass. Remember that dark glass prevents the volatile compounds of the oils from losing their efficacy. And essential oils will degrade plastic containers, possibly leaching toxins from the plastic right into your cleaning solutions.

Pets: A Word of Caution

Humans and pets respond to essential oils differently. Do not assume that what is good for you will be the equivalent (or even safe) for any animal.

It is best to consult first with a veterinarian and a trained aromatherapist before administering any essential oil for your pet's health. Essential oils have sometimes been used for dogs, horses, and some other farm animals. In these cases they have been used topically for spot application and hoof/paw care. Inhalation therapy has also been used.

As a general rule, do not use **any** essential oil topically on cats. Their metabolic systems do not break down many of the substances contained in essential oils. Liver or kidney damage, or worse, may result when cats are exposed to essential oils. This can even include exposure to essential oils via diffusion. You should use the same extreme caution with fish, reptiles, birds, rodents, and small mammals.

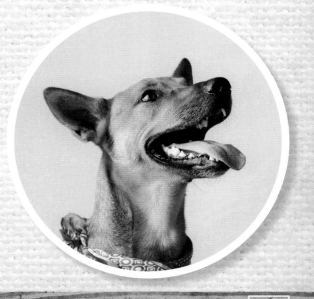

BATHROOM

The bathroom is one of the best places to use essential oils for cleaning. You'll find that tea tree and eucalyptus frequently appear in bathroom cleaning blends. They're powerful cleaners and microbe killers, they combat mold and soap residue, and they have brisk and clean aromas. But there are a number of other useful oils to consider for bathroom-specific blends, including basil, cinnamon, grapefruit, peppermint, rosemary, and thyme. And if it's cold and flu season, remember ravensara. This powerful antiviral oil can be added to your winter blends.

General Purpose Bathroom Cleaner

- 30 drops tea tree oil
- 20 drops orange oil
- 2 cups distilled water
- 2 tbsp castile soap
- 1 tbsp baking soda

Combine all ingredients in a dark glass spray bottle. When ready to use, shake bottle thoroughly and spray on problem areas. This cleaner can be used to clean or wipe up spills and residue in tubs, tiles, floors, and sinks.

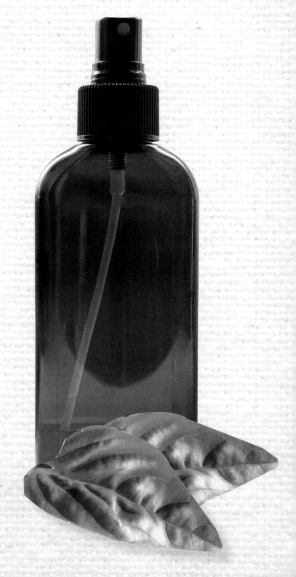

Toilet Bowl Cleaner

- —5 drops hyssop oil
- —5 drops pine oil
- —5 drops spruce oil
- —3 drops lemon oil
- —3 drops grapefruit oil
- —1 cup borax
- —1 cup white vinegar

Thoroughly stir the oils into the borax and store in a dark, airtight container. When ready to use, sprinkle several spoonfuls into toilet. Add vinegar and scrub. If possible, let mixture set in bowl overnight before scrubbing.

Soap Scum Tile Cleaner

- —10 drops eucalyptus oil
- —10 drops tea tree oil
- —5 drops lemon oil
- —5 drops orange oil
- —1 cup white vinegar

Combine all the ingredients in a dark glass spray bottle. When ready to use, shake the bottle thoroughly and spray on scummy areas and wipe clean.

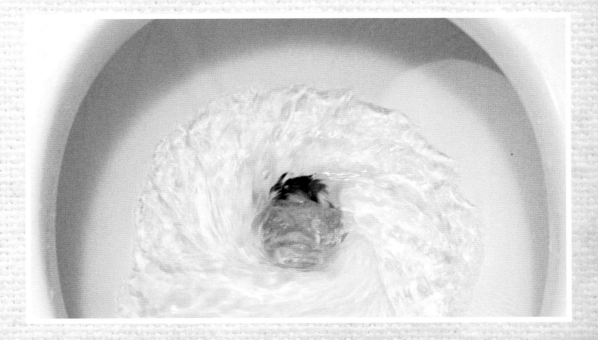

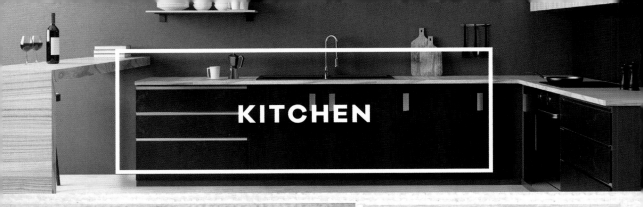

KITCHEN

If you've ever kept bananas around until they've gone bad you've met fruit flies. These pests can be tenacious. Try diffusing any of the following in your kitchen: basil, camphor, cedarwood, cypress, hinoki, rosewood, or tea tree. Studies have shown that hinoki is an especially effective repellent. You can also make a water-diluted blend from any or all of these oils and spray them directly at the flies, around the trash can, or anywhere else they might gather.

Kitchen Counter Disinfectant and Cleaner

- –5 drops cypress oil
- –5 drops grapefruit oil
- –5 drops palmarosa oil
- –5 drops rosemary oil
- –5 drops tea tree oil
- –1 cup distilled water
- –1 cup vinegar

Combine all ingredients in a dark glass container. Shake container before use. Spray on problem areas and wipe clean. (Do not use this or any vinegar-based cleaning blend on granite countertops.)

Dish Soap

- –15 drops lemon oil
- –5 drops bergamot oil
- –3 drops lavender oil
- –3 drops lime oil
- –22 ounces castile soap

Combine all ingredients in a dark glass container. Shake gently before use.

Linoleum Floor Rescue

- –3 drops clove oil
- –3 drops eucalyptus oil
- –3 drops lavender oil
- –3 drops lemon oil
- –3 drops pine oil
- –1 tablespoon castile soap
- –1 cup white vinegar
- –1 bucket hot water

Add all ingredients to a bucket of hot water and mop floor as usual.

Lemon Rosemary Glycerin Soap

- 1 pound clear glycerin soap base
- 15 drops lemon oil
- 15 drops rosemary oil
- Dried lemon peel
- Dried rosemary
- Soap molds
- Coconut oil

Prepare soap molds by greasing with coconut oil. Cut soap base into chunks, and melt in a double boiler or in the microwave (heating for 20-second intervals and stirring the soap in between intervals). Remove from heat and stir in essential oils. Place lemon peel and rosemary into soap molds, and then fill molds with soap mixture. Allow soap to set for at least two hours. Because this soap contains dried fruit and herbs, use it in a few months to prevent mold.

Tea Tree Oil Antiseptic Soap

- 2 cups clear glycerin soap base
- 2 tablespoons tea tree oil
- Soap molds
- Coconut oil

Prepare the soap molds by lightly greasing with coconut oil. Cut glycerin soap base into chunks, and then melt in a double boiler or in the microwave (heating for 20-second intervals and stirring the soap in between intervals). Remove from heat, and stir in tea tree oil. Pour into molds, and allow to set for at least two hours. Tea tree oil soap is an excellent ally to have around for cold and flu season. It's also good to have on hand to wash cuts and scrapes and protect against infection. With all of its health benefits, this is a useful soap to keep in your medicine cabinet.

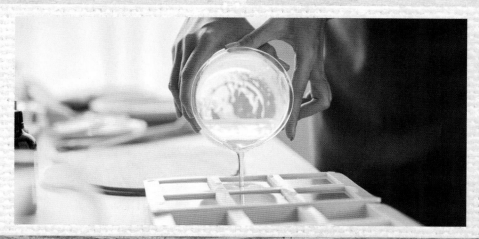

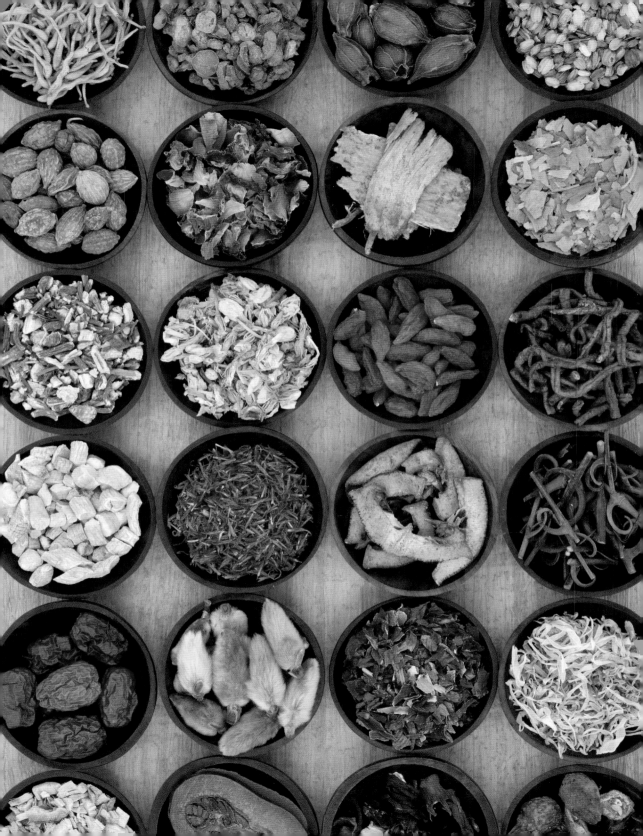